MW00948072

Soul Food

Soul Food

✦

A Dietitian's Guide to Nutritional Transformation

Terri Lykins, RD, LD

iUniverse, Inc.
New York Bloomington

Soul Food
A Dietitian's Guide to Nutritional Transformation

You should not undertake any diet/exercise regimen recommended in this book before consulting your personal physician. Neither the author nor the publisher shall be responsible or liable for any loss or damage allegedly arising as a consequence of your use or application of any information or suggestions contained in this book.

iUniverse books may be ordered through booksellers or by contacting:

iUniverse
1663 Liberty Drive, Suite 200
Bloomington, IN 47403
www.iuniverse.com
1-800-Authors (1-800-288-4677)

ISBN-13: 978-0-595-52768-7 (pbk)
ISBN-13: 978-0-595-62821-6 (ebk)

Printed in the United States of America

iUniverse Rev. 10/20/08

Contents

Acknowledgments

My sincerest thanks and appreciation to:

Father God for trusting me with this message, and guiding my steps along the way.

My parents, who raised me to believe that I am capable, resourceful, and strong, and can accomplish great things. You have been proud of me throughout the various turns of my life, and now we can see how all things work to the good for those who believe in Him. You helped me to know that I am worthy to do whatever God asks, and can do it in a manner that is well and pleasing to Him, and to you as well.

Dr. Walter Malone Jr., Founder and Pastor of Canaan Christian Church, for receiving me with open arms and immediately recognizing the value of the work that the Lord is doing in my life. Thank you for allowing me to develop this ministry with Canaan and for blessing me with an important role in the Body of our Church.

Reverend Terry Henderson, for your guidance and spiritual support. Thank you for allowing me to teach this ministry at Canaan, as a "baby Christian", knowing that the Holy Spirit had a more mature message that He wanted me to teach, and would grow me up fast with those "Holy Ghost Roller Skates" that your Grandmother described to you. Thank you to Deanna Henderson, his lovely wife, for your editorial wisdom and encouragement.

Canaan Christian Church congregation, for loving me and welcoming me from the moment I walked in the door. I have never known such a warm, kind and talented group of people, and it brings tears of appreciation to my eyes when I reflect on the joy that you bring to my life. I especially want to thank Cheryl Hammock for leading me to Canaan, and blessing me with her glorious spirit of love and acceptance. Kim Cato, I love you and appreciate your prayers and words of encouragement. Your suggestions have been very valuable and I have incorporated your ideas into this workbook.

David Evans, for extending the hand of Christ into my life, and for being my escort to Him. You inspire me in so many ways, and I will always cherish the growth, love, and laughter we share. Thank you for letting me fly in His Spirit, and go off to do His work, when the time came.

Teresa Bailey, for being my best friend in Christ, and praying me out of the spiritual warfare that was waging in my mind several years ago. I know that you were also an escort to Christ, and I value your friendship more than you will ever know.

Kathleen Hoye, thanks for standing by me and believing in my work. You always knew the best introductions to make, and are gifted at bringing people together. Tammy Spears, you are a blessing to me too, and God is moving in your life in big ways. Veronica Ballard, my dietitian school buddy, I am so pleased that God brought us back together twenty years later, so we could see what He did in our lives and allow us to walk down the path of spiritual growth together, and learn how to love ourselves as the beautiful, capable women that we are.

Preface

The information came to me so quickly, I couldn't write it fast enough. I kept a notebook on the car seat next to me and for weeks I filled the pages with concepts that burst into my mind like epiphanies. The Holy Spirit was revealing Truth to me about food and feelings in ways that I had never considered, starting with the need to change eating behavior from the inside out, rather than by applying external band-aids like surgery, diets, or pills.

He spoke to me about feeding the spirit, instead of the body, and about the deep inner hunger that only God can fill, but in our fleshly urges to self-gratify we reach for more of everything, including food.

After my notebook was filled with revelations, I created a website, www.eatwisely.org, with links about the underlying reasons why we eat, how we eat, and what we eat. These three aspects of our food relationship have been distorted by emotions, hectic lifestyles, and economics. It's easier to ignore our dysfunctional relationship with food and use a fat-blocker pill so the fried chicken won't stick to our thighs. Or, pop an herbal appetite suppressant that makes us jittery and short-tempered, but helps us avoid taking seconds at the lunch buffet. Sometimes it's an expensive year-long gym membership that we bought with the best intentions, and soon became too busy to use. All three are examples of prior personal behaviors, so I know of whence (or *wince*) I speak. Even though I am a registered dietitian, I haven't always had good eating habits.

My journey began as a girl, reading my Mother's housekeeping magazines. I loved the articles about food and dieting. In my teens, I became aware that I was slightly overweight. I read books from the school library about nutrition and weight loss, and focused on the magic word "dietitian". I thought if I became one, I would understand the mysteries of metabolism and the secrets of lifelong thinness. It didn't help that I lived to eat. I thought about food constantly, so anorexic starvation was never an option. I found it easier to track my eating throughout the day and stay between 1200-1600 calories. I lost the weight, and when the pounds did begin to creep back, I became calorie-minded again.

Spiritually, I grew up in a home with parents who had been forced to attend church when they were young and abandoned it as adults. We rarely discussed God. I did attend a Baptist church periodically with a neighborhood family for several years, but quit going as a teenager. Still, I maintained a belief in God and had questions about Christ.

I attended college and majored in dietetics, and worked for ten years as a hospital dietitian. In the evenings, I taught weight loss courses and wrote a newspaper column. In 1999, I made what was considered a strange career move by my colleagues. I was the chief dietitian at a prominent hospital, had just published an article in a major journal, and lectured nationally, when I decided to check out of all the bureaucracy to work at a holistic clinic in the middle of nowhere. It was a very well-funded clinic, so the salary was good and the benefits were extraordinary. I flew to exclusive seminars all over the country to be trained in alternative medicine. I met fascinating, intelligent, creative people who expanded my mind beyond any former dimensions. And, I was exposed to a huge dose of self-help thinking and philosophy.

In my hunger to be open-minded, I experienced everything they had to offer. Colonics, cranial-sacral treatments, dozens of varieties of massage treatments, color and sound therapies, light frequency emitters, suction cupping of the skin, far infrared sauna, tons of supplements, health foods of all shapes and flavors, medical intuitives, hypnosis, alignments, you name it. I searched for the best and most logical practices in nutrition, healing, and spirituality. I asked what I thought were deep, probing, thought-provoking questions. I dated gurus and read philosophy books. I ate organic food and slept on a water pillow, specially chosen for me by the clinic chiropractor.

When the clinic began losing money and laying people off, I opened my own office practice. I did consulting work for nursing homes, volunteered at an autism clinic, and offered weight loss classes in various locations. In recent years, I have continued my practice with an emphasis in female hormone balance, and also work with mentally retarded adults in a State hospital facility.

Through my integrated approach to nutrition, I reached the conclusion that everyone is metabolically unique and there is no one "right" diet for everyone. Percentages and types of carbohydrate, protein, and fat should be determined based on individual genetic and biochemical factors. I designed tools to help identify individual metabolic patterns so I could create custom nutrition programs for my clients. Eventually I built a computer program to do this for me. But all of the nutritional science I expounded would not translate into healthy changes unless a person wanted it. Everything I taught was so intellectualized that I felt disconnected from my clients. I was great at explaining nutrition and metabolism in simple, thought-provoking terms, and I could engage people for hours with my analogies and diagrams. But most people simply wouldn't pick up the tools I placed at their feet. Even when I wrote detailed personal menus based on all the foods they liked and told me they wanted to eat, they would follow my advice for a short time and then fall off the wagon and slip back into old habits. Sound familiar?

I had also reached a stale place in my spirituality, reading pop-culture books and constantly changing my definition of who God is, what He believes, and how He works. My personal life was becoming more focused on using food as a distraction from feelings of emptiness or a lack of motivation. I used shopping, relationships, and food to try to fill an inner void and build my self-esteem by basing my value on looking good on the outside while seeking inner comfort from food. I was sacrificing my own peace and stability by trying to acquire external validation.

So what happened to turn my life around?

I was in a new relationship with a Christian man who had an intriguing blend of conservative views mixed with artistic, musical flair and poetic creativity. One day I started interrogating him about Christianity and the Bible, two subjects I knew nothing about. I asked him tough questions about Jesus, whom I believed had historically existed and I felt was more evolved than other humans. Many say he was a prophet, and I was willing to accept that designation for Him. But the Son of God? The only way to salvation? I was too clever to think that just a simple acceptance and willingness to believe in Christ could be the answer.

During our lively discussion, I began weeping. We were both surprised by my strong emotional reaction to the conversation. I had never known anyone who I had trusted to give me straight answers about the Bible or Jesus until I met him. I knew he was too real to use dogmatic language on me.

As we talked, a huge realization struck that became my first epiphany of the Holy Spirit*: God left us an instruction manual. If I really want to know Him, I should read what He says about Himself.*

That evening, I went to church with him for the first time. I loved the contemporary Christian rock music at his church, but felt a longing for a more passionate style of worship. I started attending a smaller, more charismatic church. I grew in my enthusiasm and devotion to the Lord, and read the Bible daily. The Bible took root in me and began to assume a level of meaning and importance in my life that would have previously been impossible for me to realize or appreciate. I studied in a cell group on Thursdays, and attended Sunday worship every week. The Holy Spirit was filling me from the inside, and the insights began to flow. He spoke to me about nutrition and a deeper connection between our spirit life, emotions, thoughts, and bodies. My seeking, searching spirit finally found solid ground in the Bible, and my views about life now stood on the truth of His Word.

He revealed a diagram to me that pieced together the link between spirit, soul, and body, and the decline into unhealthy behaviors that occurs as we move farther away from the peace of the Spirit and into the fleshly appetites of the body. In the New Testament, Paul spoke of these fleshly appetites. In 1 Corinthians 6:12, he states that *everything is permissible for me; but not all things are helpful. Everything is lawful for me, but I will not become the slave of anything or be brought under its power.*

As a dietitian, I am well versed in the idea that no foods are "forbidden" and that we can and should be able to eat anything we wish, in moderation. I advocate the 80:20 guideline: Eighty percent of what we eat should be healthy and nourishing, but twenty percent can be enjoyed simply for taste pleasure. Unfortunately, when food is used for the wrong reasons, it ceases to be fun and becomes a dangerous tool of potential self-destruction. The enemy (satan) knows how to destroy us from the inside out through our own eating habits when we descend into the realm of stress relief and emotional gratification from food, rather than staying in the peace of the Spirit.

In Romans 8:5, Paul speaks about the mind of the flesh being "death". He states*: For those who are according to the flesh and are controlled by its unholy desires set their minds on and pursue those things which gratify the flesh, but those who are according to the Spirit and are controlled by the desires of the Spirit set their minds on and seek those things which gratify the Spirit.*

In verse 13, he states: *For if you live according to the dictates of the flesh, you will surely die. But if through the power of the Holy Spirit, you are habitually putting to death the deeds prompted by the body, you shall really and genuinely live forever.*

I don't read this scripture to say that we mustn't eat what we like, but that if we have strongholds that drive us to destructive overeating, we need to break free and seek to do what pleases and gratifies the Spirit. The regular effort, or *battle,* to pull down strongholds by using the weapons of our warfare as described in the Word draws us into closer intimacy with God. This intimacy creates an inner peace and joy through our close communion with Him that is intensely more powerful than the lies and false arguments of the enemy. I believe Paul is saying that we can be transformed by renewing our minds with insights and grace through our relationship with God and experience eternal peace both now and forever. This peace, that surpasses all understanding, gives us true emotional satisfaction and joy on a daily basis, which influences us to build a healthier lifestyle that begins with good eating habits. I pray that I can convey the wisdom He wishes me to provide to you in these pages, and that you experience transformation from the inside out.

He who does not use his endeavors to heal himself is brother to him who commits suicide.

(Prov 18:9)

Note: All scripture references are taken from the Amplified Bible, unless stated otherwise.

Introduction

Welcome! This book is designed to help you evaluate your own attitudes, behavior and knowledge toward food, so that you can gain insight into those eating patterns that are beneficial, and those that are destructive. After nineteen years as a practicing clinical dietitian and nutritionist, I can tell you firsthand that it isn't necessarily a lack of knowledge that locks us into destructive eating patterns leading to the plus-size department or the doctor's office. There are often spiritual, emotional, hormonal, and neurochemical (brain chemistry) factors that drive our eating behaviors in the wrong direction.

Some Christian writers denounce science and present an "either-or" approach, pitting the Bible against modern scientific discovery.

I believe that God's Word, which is the ultimate authority in all matters, is supported by science. I focus on the overlaps by putting God first, and celebrating how science creates sophisticated terminology like "*neural pathways*" to explain what the Bible has taught us for thousands of years about ***strongholds***. As modern psychologists seek ways to teach clients to reprogram their thoughts to break free of addictions and habits, we know that Paul tells us in Romans 12:2 to *be transformed by the renewing of our minds*, and scripture teaches us how to do this by *casting down imaginations, and every high thing that exalteth itself against the knowledge of God, and bringing into captivity every thought to the obedience of Christ.* (2 Cor 10:5, KJV)

Your challenge may be a stressful, demanding lifestyle that leaves you feeling helpless to find time to eat healthy as you devour your drive-thru burger and fries in the van on the way to soccer practice. It could be the sugar craving that shows up every afternoon at 3 p.m. like clockwork, resulting in a "pick me up" soda and candy bar. Maybe your hormone production is imbalanced, resulting in sugar cravings that reach far beyond the afternoon chocolate bar. I've had many patients say that they hate drinking water, and they fear the chemical effects of artificial sweeteners, so they drink regular sodas all day, which typically provide *eight teaspoons of sugar per can*. The likelihood of developing metabolic syndrome from excess sugar consumption is much greater than the risk of cancer from artificial sweeteners in acceptable daily intake (ADI) levels. Nonetheless, part of my goal as a dietitian is to educate you in options you may not know about, like Stevia, a natural non-caloric sweetener made from the leaves of the Stevia plant. And, it is available in your neighborhood grocery store, if you know where to look.

Speaking of metabolic syndrome, which usually precludes Type 2 diabetes, 23% of all Americans have this cluster of symptoms, which includes abnormal waist circumference, and elevated serum triglycerides, HDL cholesterol levels, blood pressure, and fasting blood sugar levels. This syndrome can go undetected for many years, but gradually leads to insulin resistance, weight gain and obesity, fatigue, heart disease, and/or diabetes. Despite genetic tendencies, this condition is preventable, and can be reversed with proper nutrition and exercise.

But we cannot change what we don't acknowledge and understand in ourselves. So the real benefit you obtain from this book is entirely up to you, your willingness, and your readiness to look at some potentially hard truths about your reasons for eating. No one is judging you or condemning you for your choices. If you find that you are drawn to a particular food for comfort and that food is sabotaging your health, just admitting the problem is the first step in healthy change. You will work these lessons in private, and may have the benefit of group discussion, but you are in no way obligated to reveal personal issues that you are uncomfortable sharing.

We are all unique, so there is no one right diet or nutrition plan for everyone. Just as we each have different emotional and lifestyle reasons for the food choices we make, we also vary greatly in our metabolic characteristics. Many factors influence the way our bodies use the nutrients in the food we eat, such as family history (genetics), existing medical conditions, adrenal and hormonal regulation, muscle mass, and brown adipose tissue, to name a few. There are many other components that make us each metabolically unique, and this helps explain why a diet program that works well for your neighbor may not help you at all, or could potentially make you feel worse.

This book is designed to help you identify your own physical and spiritual truths so that *you* can create a nutrition plan that will work. Not a diet, but a plan, which may include changes that go far beyond eating habits. The more honesty, open-mindedness, and willingness you bring to the table, the greater and more sustainable the benefits that you will obtain.

Now let's get started!

Getting Started

YOUR PERSONAL GOALS

Remember, there are no deadlines in reaching your health goals. You are committing yourself to writing down what you would like to become, not what your goal weight and measurements will be in a few weeks. This program involves a lifestyle change, not a quick fix. The more you pray, study God's Word, exercise, and change your eating habits, the more you will progress on this journey. Let's emphasize progress, rather than perfection!

Goal Weight____________
This may be your best weight in high school or younger adulthood, or a weight that you would feel comfortable achieving.

Calculate your Goal Weight:

Women
100 pounds for five feet tall, then add five pounds for every inch over five feet. If you have a large bone structure, add 10%; if small-boned, subtract 10%.

Men
106 pounds for five feet tall, then add six pounds for every inch over five feet. If you have a large bone structure, add 10%, if small-boned, subtract 10%.

Frame size determination: Wrap thumb and middle finger around bony part of wrist. If fingers overlap, bone frame is small. If they just touch, it is a medium frame, and if there is a gap, it is a large bone frame.

Body Measurements:

Current measurements (inches): **After the book:**

Waist________________ __________________

Hip__________________ __________________

Waist to hip ratio ________ __________________

(waist inches divided by hip inches)

Abdomen_______________ __________________

Thigh__________________ __________________

Waist to Hip Ratio (WHR) Chart		
Male	Female	Health Risk Based Solely on WHR
0.95 or below	0.80 or below	Low Risk
0.96 to 1.0	0.81 to 0.85	Moderate Risk
1.0+	0.85+	High Risk

Your health is not only affected by how much body fat you have, but also by where most of the fat is located on your body. People who tend to gain weight mostly in their hips and buttocks have roughly a pear body shape, while people who tend to gain weight mostly in the abdomen have more of an apple body shape.

If you have an apple shaped body rather than a pear shaped body, you are at increased risk for the health problems associated with obesity, such as diabetes, coronary heart disease and high blood pressure. As long as you avoid excess weight, being an apple shaped body or a pear shaped body doesn't put you at special risk - it's just one of those things to keep in mind. And even pear shaped people should take particular care to keep their weight within normal limits, to avoid the health problems associated with obesity.

My body shape is: Apple Pear (circle one)

If I reach my weight goals, I can look forward to:

____

____

____

____

____

But if we hope for what is still unseen by us, we wait for it with patience and composure. So too the Holy Spirit comes to our aid and bears us up in our weakness. (Rom 8:25-26)

The kingdom of God is not a matter of getting the food and drink one likes, but instead it is righteousness and peace and joy in the Holy Spirit. (Rom 14:17)

Yet amid all these things we are more than conquerors and gain a surpassing victory through Him Who loved us. (Rom 8:37)

Part I

In the Spirit… Getting Real About Why We Eat

We all Know the Difference Between an Apple and a Doughnut...

As a dietitian, I've spent almost two decades trying to teach people the nutritional details of food, only to see them backslide a few weeks later, and return to their former eating habits.

If knowledge alone were the key to weight control, everyone would simply memorize the calories or read the nutrition labels of the foods they regularly eat and drink, and stay within a calorie range that would maintain a perfect body weight.

For many, there is more that contributed to becoming overweight than large portion sizes or eating too many fast food meals of burgers and fries. In his book The Craving Brain, Dr. Ronald Ruden, a Harvard-trained medical nutritionist, states that among many of his overweight patients, eating when not hungry and being unable to control their food intake is a common thread. For these individuals, he says, compulsive eating was preceded by obsessive thoughts about food. He speculates that obesity is partly an obsessive-compulsive disorder that leads to increased food intake.

I found one of his statements to be very enlightening: "If this is true, it would explain current data in the weight control industry. New diet books are successful because each provides *a new obsessional focus for the hopeful buyer.* But brain-driven obsessive thoughts of food eventually override obsessive thoughts of the diet program. Non-hunger eating returns, and the weight is regained." When we focus our thoughts on battling the flesh through works-based efforts like diet rituals, we are not tearing down strongholds but reinforcing power on the enemy by drawing our focus away from God.

Take a moment to list some of the diet books and programs you have tried before:

____

____

Were you excited by the idea of totally immersing yourself in the new diet or program, only to become bored or less enthusiastic in a short time?

____

When you first started the program, did you think it was the perfect answer to your weight problems? ______________________________
Why?____

____

Were you strict about following the program? ____________________

What happened to cause you to quit? Was it a deliberate decision to stop the diet, or did you find yourself eating more than the diet allowed? __________

____

Neural Pathways

When I became a Christian, God revealed ideas and thoughts to me that I continue to investigate and unravel, with amazing results. One of the paragraphs that I wrote in my notebook of Holy Spirit nutrition revelations went like this:

> ***By the time you are an adult, you've developed some deep emotional ruts. Your emotional patterns have carved deep emotional ruts in your soul. New cars, houses, and relationships can't pull you out of those ruts for very long. Neither can a new diet book or pill. These things might change the way you feel temporarily and make you think you are getting relief, but you haven't resurfaced the road in your soul. The ruts - the faulty thinking and dysfunctional patterns - are still there, and you're going to fall right back into your old ways once the novelty of the distraction you've purchased wears off.***

The mental image I had of these "emotional ruts" was of long, straight trenches like those that would line the sides of a road. I didn't understand the significance of this image until several years later when I began to learn about *neural pathways*.

Neural pathways are lines of communication signals that the nerve cells, called neurons, send to one another. These pathways reinforce our behaviors by causing a release of feel-good brain chemicals, like dopamine, in response to certain activities. It is interesting to note that drug addiction and pleasurable food intake share the same neural pathways.

From back in the days when we were hunters and gatherers, we possessed genes that heightened sensitivity to the possibility of available food; allowed us to eat large quantities of food when it was available with weak signaling of being full; and promoted efficient storage of temporary excess calories in fat cells. This worked well when our food supply was natural and our days were long and full of physical activity.

Today, with our ready supply of fast food, vending machines and soda pop, our thrifty food genes are making us fat. In the words of one obesity researcher: "Availability of cheap calories from fat and sugar, combined with a sedentary lifestyle, are overpowering a regulatory system that was designed to deal with a scarce supply of low calorie food, frequent famines, and high physical activity" from the earlier history of our society. (Progress in Obesity Research 9. By Geraldo Medeiros-Neto, Alfredo Halpern, Claude Bouchard. Chapter 12- Neural Pathways Underlying Food Intake and Energy Homeostasis. Berthoud, Hans-Rudolf. Pg 59-63. Copyright 2003.)

Because we are hard-wired to want food frequently and to keep eating it if it is available, we must be extra careful and diligent about the food we choose to put into our bodies. Some foods cause a release of feel-good brain chemicals that reinforce us to keep eating them because we get the pleasure reward. Unfortunately, the foods that usually produce the feel-good reinforcement are sugary, salty and/or fatty foods that are synthetically created, rather than natural. Most people don't crave celery or carrot sticks when they are stressed or bored, but doughnuts, cookies or potato chips can fill the void! These are the very foods that also elevate the sugar and/or fat in our blood, putting us at increased risk of major disease. The enemy (satan) can attack our health and our spirit with poor eating habits through the neural pathways, if we allow this misuse of God's circuitry.

The carnal desires that Paul speaks of, in Corinthians, are also known to produce feel-good chemicals and to use similar neural pathways. In extreme examples, sex addictions and other forms of hedonism are reinforced by these very mechanisms.

God created our pathways and mechanisms for our own survival, and to be used for good purposes. But the enemy tries to use these same mechanisms to destroy us from within. The Biblical term for neural pathways is *strongholds.* The desire to continue beneficial or destructive activities is fueled by the release of neurotransmitters.

Consider the runners' high that some athletes experience. This is a healthy motivator to exercise, just as is the boost of serotonin that is available from doing other, less strenuous forms of exercise. Research has also shown an elevation in serotonin, an important mood-elevating neurotransmitter, from prayer.

Less desirable behaviors that can cause the release of feel-good neurotransmitters include smoking, gambling, compulsive shopping, thrill-seeking, alcoholism, drug addiction, and hundreds of other activities that may have negative consequences if taken to excess. Food can be one of those activities.

When we eat for reasons other than hunger, we need to consider our true motivation. If it is to change our mood, then we are in danger of inviting the enemy to come into our sanctuary (body) and do some damage. While the destruction may not be immediately obvious, if this pattern plays out frequently over the course of many years, we may develop heart disease, obesity, or diabetes, to name a few of the many diet-related health conditions.

My favorite special indulgence foods are:

____

____

____

Time of the day and activities I do when I eat these foods:

____

____

____

Give a recent example of a food you ate when you weren't hungry. What were you feeling when you ate the food? Stress, boredom, loneliness, fear, sadness or anxiety?

____

____

Activity: Keep a Food and Feelings journal for a few days. Record the food you eat, the time of day, and what you were feeling when you ate. Also record the activities that were going on in your life that may have contributed to how you felt, both positively and negatively.

Addressing Strongholds

> *For though we walk in the flesh, we are not carrying on our warfare according to the flesh and using mere human weapons. For the weapons of our warfare are not physical, but they are mighty before God for*

> *the overthrow and destruction of strongholds. Refute arguments and theories and reasonings and every proud and lofty thing that sets itself up against the knowledge of God; and we lead every thought and purpose away captive into the obedience of Christ. (2 Cor 10:3-5)*

Paul tells us, in Romans 12:2, not to be conformed to this world - fashioned after and adapted to its external, superficial customs - but be transformed by the renewing of your mind. The Amplified Bible further expands the text to say *be transformed (changed) by the (entire) renewal of your mind (by its new ideals and its new attitude).*

Popular culture tells us lies, like the notion that we should eat Fourth Meal at Taco Bell, which they define as that time of night when you crave their food, such as 2 or 3 am. The website they have created to justify this gluttonous behavior is very dark and creepy, with links like "Late Night Confessions" featuring a shady-looking taxi driver saying "Where were you between the hours of 10 and 2 last night? Don't worry, your secret is safe…." The website requests that you send them a video, telling what you did in the hours between dinner and breakfast, and "if your video's good enough, you just might be forgiven". The website looks and feels like a fast-food pornography site.

Fast food restaurants constantly strive to create bigger, more elaborate burgers and desserts by adding more sauce, cheese, bacon, and other fattening flavor enhancers. The message they broadcast is that we are in such a hurry with the busy demands of our life that we don't have time to think about our food so we should choose a cheap, fast, heavily flavored, salted, and fatted meal that will leave us feeling satisfied that we got our money's worth.

These false ideas create strongholds, which can be defined as *any argument or pretension that sets itself up, or exalteth itself, against the knowledge of God.* (2 Cor 10:5 various translations)

Strongholds speak lies to us from the enemy by misinforming us that a behavior or decision would make us feel better, when God's Word would have directed us otherwise. The closer we draw to God and to His Word, the better our basis for determining in our Spirit what is *helpful - good for me to do, expedient and profitable when considered with other things.* (1 Cor 6:12) The Word gets inside of us and creates a barometer against which we automatically measure all of our ideas and thoughts, when we **regularly stay in the Word**. It guides us in doing the right things and making the best choices. The world also has a barometer that is based on carnal values, and gratifying the flesh.

What are some of the false ideas and patterns we see with eating habits? Here are a few of the destructive patterns that clients have shared with me over the years. Some may seem harmless enough, but when they happen repeatedly, they take their toll, both physically and spiritually:

- Skipping breakfast, which usually results in overeating later in the day or evening
- Following restrictive diets that are based on dysfunctional eating rituals, like avoiding carbohydrates
- Eating desserts, chips, ice cream or other foods for comfort
- Stopping along the way home at multiple drive-through windows to buy and eat different foods
- Eating fast food regularly and making poor choices
- Drinking sugary sodas and/or eating candy bars in the afternoon for "energy"
- Drinking regular soft drinks for fear that diet drinks are harmful to your health
- Using diet pills and herbal supplements to suppress appetite
- Waking and eating in the middle of the night
- Not drinking enough water daily
- Rewarding or coercing your own or others' behavior with food

The first step in the overthrow and destruction of strongholds is to recognize them for what they are. There is no guilt or shame when we consider the righteousness of God that Christ died to give us. We are always susceptible to being deceived by the enemy while we are still flesh. Even Paul struggled with this, as he says in Romans 7:15: *For I do not understand my own actions. For I do not do what I want, but I do the very thing I hate.* (English Standard Version)

The solution lies in God's hands, not in focusing on our shortcomings. The goal of the list above is not to make you feel badly about your eating behaviors, but to help you identify some of your own strongholds with food so that you can gain freedom from the bondage of self by using the spiritual weapons of our warfare.

What are some of the strongholds you have identified in your eating behaviors?

____

____

____

____

____

____

> *Whereas she who lives in pleasure and self-gratification is dead, even while she still lives. (1 Tim 5:6)*
>
> *Let no one say when he is tempted, "I am being tempted by God," for God cannot be tempted with evil, and He Himself tempts no one. But each person is tempted when he is lured and enticed by his own desire. (Jas 1:13-14 ESV)*

The Pulling Down of Strongholds

Scripture defines strongholds as *arguments and every pretension that sets itself up against the knowledge of God.* We generally consider strongholds to be patterns of behaviors and beliefs that steal our focus and cause us to feel overwhelmed, or even powerless to change. The enemy lies to us through strongholds and deceives us into believing that the stronghold is bigger than God. That we need this behavior or thought to compensate for a void in our life that God can't fill. That it is okay to have this one little pleasure if we are doing the rest of our Christian walk properly. That we needn't be overly rigid about our lives. After all, it's my body. Who cares if I want to splurge sometimes?

When we place a harmful behavior, thought, or belief ahead of our reliance upon God, it can become a stronghold. In the Old Testament, the word "stronghold" was synonymous with "fortress". When we consider how a stronghold sets itself up against the knowledge of God, we can picture it blocking the influence of the Holy Spirit (Truth) by creating a fortress around an erroneous (false) thought pattern.

The Word arms us with weapons that are *mighty for the overthrow and destruction of strongholds* (2 Cor 10:4). Scripture guides us through the steps of deliverance from these harmful patterns by bringing our thoughts into submission to Christ. The battlefield is in the mind. As we wage this war, remember that *we are not wrestling with flesh and blood, but against the despotisms, against the powers, against the world rulers of this present darkness, against the spiritual forces of wickedness in the heavenly sphere.* (Eph 6:12)

Consider the word *despotism.* The definition is "a government or political system in which the ruler exercises absolute power; or the state that exists when one person or group has power over another". The enemy claims power over our minds when we are deceived into believing that we need a food, behavior, person, activity or substance more than we need God, to be content or satisfied. Please don't confuse the basic need for food when we are hungry with a food stronghold. Hunger is a healthy physical need. Food strongholds relate to a different form of hunger, a soul hunger that creates a longing to fill a hole inside that only God can fill.

How can we approach a process of pulling down strongholds? Consider the following steps, which we will amplify through scripture and discussion:

- See it
- Confess it
- Rebuke it
- Release it
- Bind it

See It: Becoming Aware of Strongholds

Some of the patterns that can signal compulsive overeating strongholds:

- You eat when you are angry or bored
- You eat for comfort in times of tension or crisis
- You lie to yourself or others about how much you have eaten
- You hide food away for yourself
- Significant people in your life have expressed concern about your eating patterns
- Your weight has fluctuated by more than ten pounds in the past six months
- You fear that your eating is out of control

A yes answer to several of these questions can indicate strong compulsions to overeat. You may identify more easily with the eating behaviors that are listed on page 13, but regardless of the severity of the patterns, they are working against your desire for a healthy body as a temple for your Christian life. These patterns rob you of the energy and vitality needed to live your life to the fullest, and to fulfill the mission that God has for you to accomplish.

List the top three food strongholds that you recognize in yourself:

____

____

Circle the behaviors that may represent a possible stronghold:

✓ My Aunt made Chess pie, and I wanted a piece after supper, even though I ate a big meal and I wasn't really hungry.

✓ I daydream about what I will eat after Church and have trouble focusing on Pastor's sermon, week after week.

✓ Occasionally I get the desire to eat fast food French fries or a burger, and I allow myself to have this as a treat a few times a month.

✓ I don't have time to fix breakfast, so each morning I go to the vending machine and I get a pack of oatmeal cookies.

✓ I eat a very low carbohydrate diet every day and this is the only way I can lose weight, nothing else has ever worked.

✓ When Girl Scout cookie season comes along, I always order a few boxes. I have to admit, when I start eating them it is hard to stop, and sometimes I will eat almost a whole box in one evening.

Notice the aspects of these statements that indicate potential strongholds. It isn't the occasional behaviors, but the patterns that play out repeatedly in our lives that lead to cumulative destruction that serves the enemy, not God. Underline the words in the above statements that indicate stronghold patterns.

There is another form of food stronghold, which is steeped in denial. This is seen in people who pay no attention to their portion sizes and have no consideration for the high calorie, fat and sugar content of their daily diet. These folks may feel that it just doesn't matter what they eat or how much weight they gain. It may serve as their defense and protection against relationships or intimacy. This sometimes originates from abusive relationships with the opposite sex, but not always. It can be very hard to see and admit this type of stronghold in oneself, but the first step toward healing and obtaining freedom from this pain is to see the truth of the situation. The enemy hates it when we expose his lies to the light of the Truth.

> *And those who belong to Christ Jesus have crucified the flesh with its passions and appetites and desires. (Gal 5:24)*

Search me, O God, and know my heart! Try me and know my thoughts! And see if there is any wicked or hurtful way in me, and lead me in the way everlasting. (Ps 139:23-24)

Note that in the above scripture, *the hurtful way in me* can refer not only to hurtfulness we have toward others, but also toward ourselves. Consider this scripture:

Do you not know that your body is the temple of the Holy Spirit Who lives within you, Whom you have received from God? You are not your own. You were bought with a price. So then, honor God and bring glory to Him in your body. (1 Cor 6:19-20)

Confess it: Calling out the Strongholds

Now that we have become aware of our food strongholds, we can take action toward freedom and victory, based on the directive found in James 5:16 which states:

Confess to one another therefore your faults and pray for one another, that you may be healed and restored (to a spiritual tone of mind and heart). The earnest prayer of a righteous man makes tremendous power available.

And based on the words of David in Psalm 32, verse 5:

I acknowledged my sin to You, and my iniquity I did not hide. I said, I will confess my transgressions to the Lord (continually unfolding the past till all is told) then You forgave me the guilt and iniquity of my sin. Selah!

Two simple but powerful directives - confess your strongholds (false beliefs or pretensions that set themselves up against the knowledge of God) to God, and to another person. This action is powerful in helping to renew our minds by our first becoming aware of the strongholds, then telling them to God and to a trusted friend. This takes power away from the false belief or pretense, and acknowledges God's authority over every area of our lives. In this way, the strongholds begin to lose their strength and grip on our minds and our lives, and they become weak grasps.

As you enter into a prayerful state with God, take a moment to reflect on the strongholds you have identified. State them out loud to acknowledge them to the Lord. It is important to follow this with prayer based on God's Word, such as is found in 1 John 1:9. An example prayer might sound like this:

"Father, I recognize that I have strongholds in my eating behaviors. I want to be free of the desire to eat sweets and desserts in the evenings because I am lonely, and frustrated at my job. I confess that I have been trying to take my comfort from food instead of turning to You, Father God. I know that you have told us that if we freely admit that we have sinned and confess our sins, You are faithful and just and will forgive our sins and cleanse us from all unrighteousness."

The next step is to discuss the stronghold behaviors with a trusted friend or church advisor. The goal is to share honestly and to seek prayer from a fellow disciple in the Body of Christ. James 5:16 speaks of the power available to us from the earnest prayer of a righteous man. Do not be embarrassed to share honestly with this person and then ask them to pray with you. James 4:6-7 states:

> *God resists the proud, but gives grace to the humble. Therefore submit to God. Resist the devil and he will flee from you. (New King James version)*

It is interesting to note that one of the key steps of 12-step recovery programs, like Alcoholics Anonymous, is based on similar spiritual principles. Step Five states: "We admitted to God, to ourselves, and to another human being the exact nature of our wrongs." The twelve steps have helped thousands of alcoholics and compulsive overeaters to recover. As Christians, we have more power than this through scripture, which will actually draw us closer to Him, through obedience to His Word:

> *Yet amid all these things we are more than conquerors and gain a surpassing victory through Him Who loved us. (Rom 8:37)*

Christ died so that we could have full, complete lives with the Holy Spirit dwelling in us. We are His children - heirs of God and fellow heirs with Christ. If we walk and live in the Spirit, Paul tells us we will certainly not gratify the cravings and desires of the flesh. The fruit of the Holy Spirit - the work which His presence within us accomplishes - is love, joy, peace, patience, kindness, goodness, faithfulness, gentleness, and self-control. When these qualities are activated in us, we find an inner peace that does not cry out for cookies, or other external fixes, to bring us true joy. We already have it through Him.

Rebuke it: Taking Authority over Strongholds in Jesus' Name

The definition of the word "rebuke", which is used in the Old and New Testaments, is to criticize or reprove sharply; reprimand.

When Jesus and his disciples were in the boat, a sudden and violent storm came upon the sea. He continued to sleep, but the disciples were scared that they would perish.

They awakened Him, saying "Lord, rescue and preserve us! We are perishing!"

> *And He said to them, "Why are you timid and afraid, O you of little faith?" Then He got up and rebuked the winds and the sea, and there was a great and wonderful calm. And the men were stunned with bewildered wonder and marveled, saying, "What kind of Man is this, that even the winds and the sea obey Him!" (Mt 8:25-27)*

Christ wasn't intimidated by the natural events and turmoil around Him. He had power over the winds and the sea, and knew that they would not crush Him. He called them down by rebuking them, and they ceased to create fear for the disciples.

We need to take our full authority, in Christ Jesus, to banish the stronghold from our thoughts and our lives by rebuking it - telling it to leave our mind, and that it has no claim on our lives. James 4:6 tells us that *He gives us more and more grace, or power of the Holy Spirit, to meet this evil tendency and all others fully.*

Strongholds may look menacing, and engulf us in the desire to act upon them, much like the storm the disciples feared. We may feel swallowed in the waves of desire to eat something unhealthy over and over, or return to an unhealthy relationship again.

We need to rebuke - to chastise, scold, reprimand, pick apart, and correct the stronghold, to further loosen its grip. We might say something like this: "This behavior I have been acting upon in the evenings, feeling like I have to eat cookies at night before I go to bed, is just plain wrong. I don't want this, need this, or believe this nonsense anymore. This behavior is making me gain weight, it is raising my blood sugar, and it is keeping me in bondage. With the authority I have over lies and sin through Christ Jesus, I rebuke this behavior and banish it from my life. Greater is He who lives in me than He who is in the world."

The battlefield is in the mind, which influences our emotions, and our will. The soul, or personality of each of us, is made up of these three components: Mind, Emotions, and Will. Consider the following diagram:

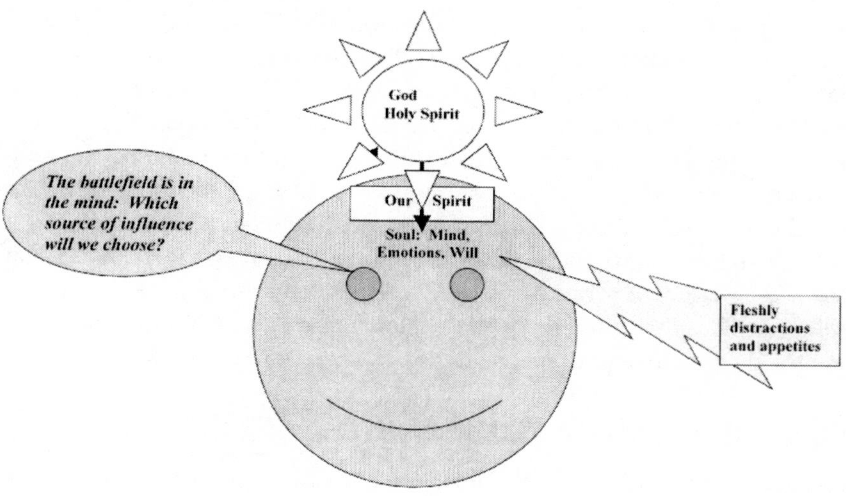

Diagram 1

God, as the Holy Spirit, influences us to know Truth and to make good lifestyle choices that are nourishing to our soul and body. But the enemy tries to speak to our soul through the flesh. If we allow the flesh to influence our choices and decisions, these will gratify the body only, and will not serve the Spirit. Paul says in Romans 8, verse 6: *Now the mind of the flesh is death, but the mind of the Spirit is life and peace, both now and forever.* In verse 9, he continues, *but you are not living the life of the flesh, you are living the life of the Spirit, if the Spirit of God dwells within you. But if anyone does not possess the Spirit of Christ, he is none of His.*

These two influences are constantly competing in our mind, to guide our emotions and our actions:

> *If we walk and live habitually in the Holy Spirit, by being responsive to, controlled, and guided by the Spirit, then we will certainly not gratify the cravings and desires of the flesh. For the desires of the flesh are opposed to the Holy Spirit, and the desires of the Spirit are opposed to the flesh; these are antagonistic to each other - continually withstanding and in conflict with each other - so that you are not free but are prevented from doing what you desire to do.*
> (Gal 5:16-17)

In Mark 7:17-23, Jesus explained to the disciples that what goes into a man from the outside cannot make him unhallowed or unclean. He used food as His example, explaining that it does not reach and enter a person's heart, but only his digestive tract, and so passes on. Thus he was making and declaring all foods clean. It isn't the food itself that is the problem, any more than anything else that "tempts" us in the world and in the flesh. The flesh doesn't have the power to make us sin, or do anything harmful to ourselves or others. We may be triggered to want something from what we see, but it is the thoughts (mind) and feelings (emotions) that we act upon (will) that determine what comes out of us (body). If we have an impure thought or feeling, we have the ability through the Holy Spirit and the Word to take that thought away captive into the obedience of Christ and cut it off.

Release it: Free Your Mind

We immediately move into the next step, which is to RELEASE IT. We ask God to keep us free from this stronghold, and we turn our will and our lives over to His care. If we are waging this warfare on a stronghold concerning a person, or a relationship, we imagine releasing the person to God. We know that God has the power to change us, through the Holy Spirit, and to help us to be free if we sincerely desire to please Him and operate in His grace.

Once we release the stronghold, it is very important that we wear the whole armor of God at all times, to protect ourselves from further attack. Be prepared, because the enemy doesn't like it when we gain freedom from strongholds. We may discover that another area of our lives becomes more problematic, like our money spending or our computer internet surfing. Recent studies have shown that persons undergoing gastric bypass surgery to lose weight often develop addictions in other directions, such as gambling and compulsive shopping. The term for this is *addiction transference.*

Go to Ephesians 6:14-18. Fill in the following information about the protective armor that we are to wear:

The belt of ________________
The breastplate of ________________________
Shod your feet with ______________________________________
The shield of ____
The helmet of ____
The sword which is the __________________ of God

Which of the above is an actual weapon? Which are defensive components?

____

____

____

____

How does this passage instruct us in the use of the shield of saving faith?

____

____

____

____

____

In Galatians 5:24, Paul tells us that those who belong to Christ Jesus have crucified the flesh with its passions, and appetites, and desires. Crucifixion is a painful death of deprivation. Hunger and thirst are present, but the lack of oxygen reaching the lungs can ultimately lead to death by suffocation. Compare this to crucifying the *flesh*, which is described in the Amplified Bible as the Godless human nature. If we suffocate and give no breath and nourishment to the carnal appetites, passions and desires, they will eventually be lifted from us, as we experience deliverance. But we must remain diligent and stand ready to resist and bind these strongholds over and over again, until they are history!

Bind it: Wrap it Tight With Scripture so it Cannot Move in Your Life Any More!

Jesus told the disciples, in Matthew 16:19, "*I will give you the keys of the kingdom of heaven, and whatever you bind (declare to be improper and unlawful) on earth must be what is already bound in heaven; and whatever you loose (declare lawful) on earth must be what is already loosed in heaven.*"

Once we release a stronghold, we can prevent its' reestablishment by binding it. This once-powerful stronghold is now becoming downgraded to a less powerful, but unwanted, thought or purpose.

Going back to 2 Corinthians 10:4-5 concerning strongholds, Paul states that *we refute arguments and theories and reasonings and every proud and lofty thing that sets itself up against the knowledge of God; and we lead every thought and purpose away captive into the obedience of Christ.*

Paul drew a distinction in this verse between the arguments, theories, reasonings, and proud and lofty things - the characteristics of strongholds - and the precursors of strongholds, which are the thoughts and purposes that we can lead away captive unto the obedience of Christ, before we act on our thoughts/purposes and activate them to become potential strongholds.

We have to lead our thoughts away captive unto the obedience of Christ because our minds are undisciplined. If you want to discipline a child, you deal with their behaviors. When dealing with the mind, we approach our thoughts as we do the behaviors of a child. If you can stop the behaviors of a child early, you can keep a pattern from forming. Make your thoughts behave Christ and the Word. Undisciplined thoughts that anchor in, and are fertilized through action, develop roots. The roots can develop offshoots to other undesirable behavior patterns, so that when one behavior is cut off, others crop up.

Each and every time the craving or desire to engage in a destructive behavior crops up, we can lead it away captive into the obedience of Christ by using scripture to bind it. A simple example prayer: *I have victory over this matter and will not be led astray. I am a new creation in Christ, the old has passed away. Behold, the fresh and new has come!* (2 Cor 5:17)

Picture what happens if you were to bind a person to a stake. One wrap of the rope wouldn't be enough to keep them from wriggling around and possibly even breaking free. But each successive wrap of the rope binds them tighter and tighter, until there is nothing that they can move freely. Each time an unwanted thought might creep back into our minds, we use our will to resist the enemy's bait by binding it with scripture. As an added bonus, this diligent prayer and scripture-speaking draws us closer to God, which really puts the enemy in his place!

Keep in mind that this is a process, not a destination. We will have to deal with unwanted thoughts and behaviors throughout our time in the flesh, but we have powerful tools and authority in Christ to be victorious over all things.

I can do all things through Christ who strengthens me. (Phil 4:13, World English Bible translation)

PART II

In the Soul... How the Mind, Emotions and Will Influence the Way We Eat

Did you know that there are dozens of nerve chemicals (neurotransmitters) and hormones that regulate your appetite and even influence the types of foods you desire? A hormone is a substance originating in an organ, gland or other part of the body that is sent through the blood to another part of the body, and stimulates it by a chemical action to increase function or secretion. There are many different categories of hormones. A hormone or neurotransmitter imbalance can cause weight and appetite problems, stress, mood disorders, and sleep disturbances. Cortisol, for example, is a stress hormone that increases fat intake. Oxytocin reduces salt cravings. Norepinephrine increases your desire to eat sweets, as does a low serotonin level. Most neurotransmitters are manufactured in the brain, but some are created from proteins that are part of your diet intake.

Your blood sugar levels and stress levels help regulate appetite and can contribute to the release of hormones that can influence your mood, and food-seeking behavior. This is why it is so important that what you eat supports the proper balance of energy, hormone, and brain chemical production, so you can feel your best and radiate the joy of the Lord to others. You don't need to understand biochemistry to catch the take-home message here. It is really very simple: Eat a healthy balance of good quality carbohydrate, protein and fat, starting with breakfast. In the third section of this book, you will learn about the best types of carbohydrates, what foods are good protein sources, and which fats are healthy and can decrease inflammation in the body. But before we get into the nuts (yes, they're healthy!) and bolts of WHAT specifically to eat, which is in the realm of the *body*, we need to be really clear about the factors that affect HOW we choose our food (soul).

Kingdom Order Versus World Order

What are the factors that drive our eating habits? In the first section of this book, we took time to understand the spiritual realm in regard to the eating behaviors that were creating strongholds in our lives. We took stock of the destructive patterns and *cleaned house.* As we continue that work, we need to now focus on the soul, which houses the mind, emotions, and will. Disturbances at this level give the enemy a doorway to walk through and to wage an attack that could result in stronghold formation. The issues that affect our eating patterns in the soul include body chemistry, lifestyle, attitudes toward food, and awareness of the consequences attached to our choices in what we eat. It is also important to address overall emotional disturbances in this area, too.

The world teaches us to view ourselves in a holistic order that is body, soul, and spirit. The body is given top priority. The philosophy is: What we see and do in the flesh (body) influences what we think and feel (soul), which eventually reaches our spirit, viewed as an ethereal, intangible aspect of oneself. The mindset is "what I see changes what I think about who I am". Behaviorally, the message is that "until I *act* good (body), I can't *think* (soul or mind) that I *am* (spirit) good". (Don Blevins, Foundations for Successful Living: Righteousness, © 2006.) This is works-based mentality. This is one reason why rigid diets that tell you what to eat and what not to eat don't work. The works-based concept is that if I am a "good girl" and follow the rules of the diet, I will be rewarded with weight loss and be a better person. This is externally driven, trying to correct us from the outside-in. Strict rules that govern eating patterns are not going to change the root of the problem, which lies in the soul. Diagram 1 on page 19 illustrates that the attempts to change the soul through the body can be enemy-driven. We need to put the spirit first, and let the Holy Spirit within us be the Lord and Influencer of our will, our thoughts, and our emotions.

The Kingdom Order:

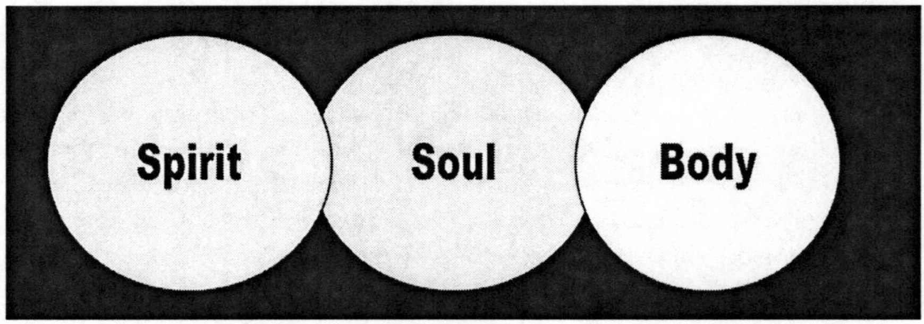

Diagram 2

This order shows us that who we are is determined by our spirit, not our body. When we are saved, the nature of God is deposited in us. The glory of God in our spirit needs to rule our soul and flow out through our body. This right way of seeing ourselves tells us that who we are in our spirit changes what we think, opening our soul up to release our nature into our body and manifest the glory of God into the Earth.

This order assures us that receiving the Holy Spirit through accepting Christ as our personal Lord and Savior changes who we are, which changes what we do. God sanctifies us spirit, soul and body. He starts with our spirit, not our body. Jesus stated, in John 3:6, *"what is born of flesh is flesh, and what is born of the Spirit is spirit."*

Once we accept Jesus Christ into our lives, the Holy Spirit enters our life to start transforming us through progressive sanctification. We begin to view the world, people, and personal difficulties from a more biblical perspective. Our choices begin to be motivated by love and truth instead of selfishness. We move from being takers to becoming givers, through the overflowing of Spirit moving out of us and into the world. The transformation process may be painful, but it is always motivated by God's love for us.

The word **transformation** is very important in this context. Paul appealed to the Romans not to *be conformed to this world, being fashioned after and adapting to its external, superficial customs, but be* ***transformed*** *by the entire renewal of your mind.* (Rom 12:2)

Conforming occurs by outside pressure and force bearing upon us to follow socially accepted standards, conventions, rules, or laws. Transformation, however, is an inside job. The metamorphosis of a caterpillar into a butterfly has often been used to illustrate the principle of transformation that we are considering. The caterpillar doesn't conform to what the world expects it to be, and therefore acts like a butterfly. Instead, the caterpillar undergoes a gradual series of changes, where is eats and grows until it is too big for its skin, and grows a new skin underneath the outer skin, which it molts, or sheds, when it is ready. It does this five times, with a final molting that is quite different. When the caterpillar molts for the fifth and final time, the new skin underneath forms the outer shell of the **chrysalis.** The chrysalis (generically referred to as a pupa), is not a "resting" stage as many people think. Quite to the contrary, a lot is happening to the pupa. The body of the caterpillar is transforming into an adult butterfly! Wings are fully formed in the chrysalis. Antennae are formed, and the chewing mouthparts of the caterpillar are transformed into the sucking mouthparts of the butterfly. After 10-14 days in the chrysalis, the butterfly is ready to emerge. (from www.butterflyschool.org

These changes were hidden from view, but they resulted in a powerful transformation within the caterpillar.

As we undergo the transformation that occurs by renewing our minds, it is important to clear away the emotional wreckage of the past, where there is anger, fear, anxiety, guilt, remorse, shame, or other negative emotions. Our emotions stem from our thoughts, and scripture tells us what to think about.

Philippians 4:8 tells us to focus on *whatever is true, whatever is worthy of reverence and is honorable and seemly, whatever is just, whatever is pure, whatever is lovely and lovable, whatever is kind and winsome and gracious, if there is any virtue and excellence, if there is anything worthy of praise, think on and weigh and take account of these things*. Paul tells us that if we do this, *the God of peace (of untroubled, undisturbed well-being) will be with you.* (Phil 4:9)

What are some examples of changes that we try to make in ourselves by conforming to the world's standards?

____

____

____

Will you stay changed permanently by adopting new eating patterns based on what someone else tells you to do?

____

____

What would have to occur before the knowledge of helpful and harmful eating habits would really result in a difference in your choices?

____

____

____

____

> *So whoever cleanses himself will be a vessel, set apart and useful for honorable and noble purposes, consecrated and profitable to the Master, fit and ready for any good work. (2 Tim 2:21)*
>
> *Woe to you, scribes and Pharisees, pretenders! For you clean the outside of the cup and of the plate, but within they are full of extortion and grasping self-indulgence. You blind Pharisee! First clean the inside of the cup and of the plate, so that the outside may be clean also. Woe to you, scribes and Pharisees! For you are like tombs that have been whitewashed, which look beautiful on the outside but inside are full of dead men's bones and everything impure. (Mt 23:25-27)*

Clearing Away Emotional Wreckage

We may be holding onto past hurts and feelings of anger, frustration, fear, anxiety or sadness when we think of certain things. The feelings can come about when we think about some people, or places we've worked or lived, institutions or agencies, like the IRS, or even things like the neighbor's loud car, or the short lunch break that doesn't seem to allow enough time to eat and return phone calls. The key is that we feel these emotions each time these things come to our thoughts. This emotional baggage is holding us back, and hindering our transformational process. Why is this important to a book about nutrition?

Because the spirit and soul need to be filled with God's inspiration and influence in order to reduce stress, improve well-being, and keep the neurotransmitters and hormones flowing in line with health. The best diet in the world won't protect you from heart disease and other maladies if you are "stewing in your own juices", to quote a nurse I once worked with, years ago. I have since forgotten her name, but her wise words continue to be validated, as we better understand the harmful release of body chemicals, like adrenaline, that are produced during stress. You may not think it is stressful to have hurt feelings or to dislike certain people who you think have wronged you, but this negative mindset takes you out of being a giving, generous, FORGIVING soul to being critical, negative, bitter and otherwise unpleasant. Consider the following diagram:

SELFLESS	***SELFISHNESS***

Giver

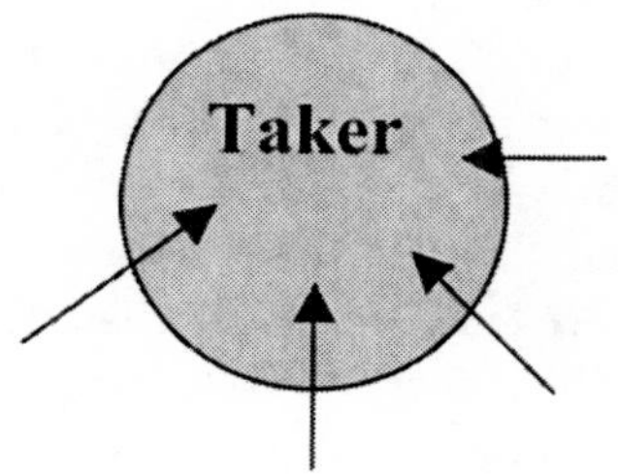

Operates from the inside-out	Operates from the outside-in
Cup is filled, gives from overflow	Bottomless pit, never satisfied
Motives: Helping others	Self-gratification, seeking to alter or change mood, motivated by feelings
Actions: Listening, considering, focusing on others' ideas and feelings without regard for self-benefit	Focusing on self, trying to dominate conversation, topics, discussion for self-benefit

What can I *bring to* the situation? Emotions: Grateful, blessed, fulfilled, enthusiastic, joyful, energetic, satisfied, pleased, completeness, fullness, PEACE	What can I *take from* the situation? Needy, wanting, restless, lacking, entitled to but not getting, unfair, left out, unsatisfied, missing out, seeking, searching for gratification
	Can descend into: lust, carnality, greed, corruption, demanding, risk-taking, thrill-seeking, abusive to self or others
Reliance upon God Spirit-filled	Reliance upon mammon Flesh-based
ABUNDANCE	NEED

Diagram 3

Most people will fluctuate on a continuum between these two models, but the ideal is on the left, and the reality of life when driven by the appetites of the flesh is on the right. We all recognize the extreme examples of a selfish life in people who do unspeakable things like abandoning their children, having multiple families in various cities, stealing their elderly parent's pain medications for their own drug addiction, and so forth. But what about the more subtle forms of selfishness? Have you known anyone who felt that she had to buy the latest $400 designer handbag, only to realize a few days later that she needed equally attractive matching shoes, too? Maybe the kids or the creditors had to wait a little longer to get what they wanted, as a result. Or people who moan that they bought a larger house in a nicer neighborhood, and their old furnishings just weren't good enough any more? The bottomless pit of materialism leads to debt, disappointment, and financial ruin. Worse, as we continue to value and define ourselves by material standards, we elevate our stress levels and are more susceptible to destructive eating behaviors and other mood-altering activities. The flesh gets hungrier and hungrier.

So how can we address the emotional hurts and resentments that we wish for God to heal in us? First, we need to recognize them. One way is to write a list of people, places and things about which we have anger, frustration or other painful feelings. We pray for the Holy Spirit to show us these things, and take notes as we are shown these disturbances.

After we make our list, we consider it from the standpoint that sometimes the world and the people around us can hurt us, without even meaning to do so. We pray and ask God to show us our part in these situations, so that we can grow and become better able to handle life from a perspective of understanding, versus demanding. We consider what was hurt in ourselves by the situation - was it our pride, ego, ambitions, or personal relationships? We write this down, so we can review this from a different perspective than before.

Finally and most importantly, we pray to apply **forgiveness** to each situation, person, place or thing. Though it doesn't change the wrongs done to us, the Divine blessing of forgiveness is like a healing balm to the soul. In the flesh, we tend to think that we are owed apologies, and want to see a change of behavior before we are willing to forgive. AREN'T YOU GLAD THAT GOD DIDN'T TREAT US THAT WAY! While we were yet sinners, Christ died for us. God made the ultimate sacrifice for us, without us having to earn it. Praise you, Lord!

Jesus taught us to practice forgiveness toward our enemies and others who we feel have wronged us:

> *You have heard that it was said, You shall love your neighbor and hate your enemy; But I tell you, Love your enemies and pray for those who persecute you.* (Mt 5:43-44)

And when Christ taught us to pray, in the Lord's Prayer, He said, *and forgive us our debts, as we also have forgiven our debtors.* (Mt 6:12)

As situations arise in your life, moving forward, try to put yourself in the other person's place. God certainly put Himself in our place, on the cross. Consider what the other person may be feeling, rather than believing that what is happening is all about you. I had a situation arise at work recently, and it helped me to talk through the circumstances with a Christian co-worker. I was feeling slighted over not being included in a project as much as I thought I should have been. I even wondered if I was intentionally excluded. Then I took a step back and began describing what may be happening, from the other person's perspective, if I were to give her the benefit of the doubt. Before long, I understood that the person was enthusiastic about her part of the project, and because I was there only a few days a week, she moved ahead full steam. It wasn't about me! It was much easier then to let go of the frustration and to pray that if I needed to say something about it at some point, God would keep me in a peaceful place where I would not be confrontational, but understanding of her feelings.

Forgiveness may not mean much to the other person, but **we** are the real benefactors. Forgiveness blesses us, regardless of anyone else. Each time you re-feel those negative feelings, you invite the enemy into your emotions and thoughts. This increases the likelihood of reaching for a quick fix, to change your stress and body chemistry. These fixes include food! This is why we must be free on all levels in order to be nourished completely from spirit to soul, and body.

And may the God of peace Himself sanctify you through and through; and may your spirit and soul and body be preserved sound and complete and found blameless at the coming of our Lord Jesus Christ. (1 Thess 5:23)

Forgiving and Loving Ourselves: God Does, Why Shouldn't We?

The world tries to tell us how we should look, speak, dress, act, think, eat, and live. The standards we are given for appearance are damaging to our spirit and soul, if we accept these messages as truth.

> Jesus tells us not to *judge, criticize and condemn others, so that you may not be judged and criticized and condemned yourselves. For just as you judge and criticize and condemn others, you will be judged and criticized and condemned, and in accordance with the measure you use to deal out to others, it will be dealt out again to you.* (Mt 7:1-2)

As we practice forgiveness and love toward others, we quickly see that we must stop judging other people and be quick to give them the benefit of the doubt. But how often do we treat ourselves this way? Do we condemn ourselves for an appearance that by Hollywood standards is less than perfect?

The pressure on us to be thin and have certain types of features is damaging. There is no true standard of beauty except that which God describes for our inner man or woman, being led by the Spirit. The inner radiance that the Holy Spirit produces within us is stunning and engaging; it is an enduring beauty. The world's standard is not based in Truth, but in superficial distortions that are driven by lust of the flesh.

When we stop judging and valuing others by their external ability to conform to the world's standards of beauty, we will stop judging ourselves this way. The Holy Spirit radiating out of a person is the most beautiful transformer of appearance that we can behold. The Spirit in me can see the Spirit in you, and that makes us lovely to one another regardless of our skin color, hairstyles, clothes, or other external characteristics. Our inner character can discern that beauty immediately. When we see others with a Spirit-filled eye, we value the characteristics we see that uphold the standards we receive through God, and are saddened when we see someone who is trying to find value by cheapening their appearance to gain approval.

The enemy can use self-doubt about our appearance to elevate our stress hormones, like adrenaline and cortisol, and motivate us toward mood-altering, destructive behaviors with food, relationships, overspending, drinking, and the like. The distractions of the world are constantly competing for the attention of our mind. If we fill our time worrying about our perceived shortcomings and trying to change our hair, clothes, makeup, and other external factors, we are digging the hole in our soul deeper. The bottomless pit can't be filled with these things. There is nothing wrong with trying to look our best, but when we are constantly focused on this as a means of trying to make peace with ourselves and gain the approval of others, it can be destructive. It channels our resources away from the things of God and onto the things of the flesh. Think about the difference between moderation and obsession. We can enjoy worldly things in moderation, without having to experience their destructiveness. When their pursuit becomes a drive, we are stepping into the dangerous realm of strongholds and obsessive behavior.

As we turn away from the world and the grip it has had on our thoughts and our feelings, we continue to mix together a healing balm of forgiveness, awareness of what is helpful and what is not, a desire to please God, and repentance. The transformational effect of the balm, when applied with God's healing touch, is acceptance and love of self and others, freedom from the bondage of our emotional baggage, and peace of the spirit that surpasses all understanding.

By experiencing inner peace, and love of ourselves and others, we lose interest in temporarily following trendy diets for the sake of losing weight to gain others' approval. We value ourselves so much that we want to be healthy and take care of ourselves, which includes removing destructive eating behaviors and other tendencies that work against our ability to advance God's kingdom on Earth.

What will lead you to lasting change? It won't happen by trying to be someone different on the outside, but by loving yourself and seeing yourself as the beautiful person you are in Christ. Self-love will keep you from destroying yourself, and cause you to care about what you eat and the effect it will have upon your body, your mood, and your health.

Many Americans love their pets more than they love themselves. We don't wait for our pets to behave a certain way, or look cute enough, to feed, walk, and care for them. We tend to the things we love and treat them well. Let's do the same for ourselves, without saying "I'll eat well when I find time", or "I'll exercise when I lose twenty pounds." Let's learn how to take care of something that we love – ourselves - so that we can also nourish the Christ nature within us. The radiant beauty and light that shines as a result will lead others to the Kingdom, as they are mysteriously attracted to His presence in us.

Suggested activity: Watch the short documentary (7 minutes long) entitled "A Girl Like Me", by Director Kiri Davis. This film can be viewed online at www.mediathatmattersfest.org by typing the title of this film in the "search" box on the home page.

Pulling It All Together

Let's take a moment to consider the different components of the spirit, soul and body that we have discussed so far, and how they influence each other. Diagram 4 shows that there are external, situation-based triggers that can activate deep-seated negative emotions in our soul. These include financial problems, relationship or health issues, and other troubles that may occur in life. They touch at our fears and insecurities, which may activate the release of stress compounds in our bodies.

Internal triggers are based on hormones, blood sugar, neurotransmitters and other physiological compounds that the body attempts to regulate and if imbalanced, can generate stress. Stress motivates us to engage in behavior(s), which may include overeating, to change our internal chemistry by producing feel-good compounds so that we are content again. If we choose to turn to God and the Word, we strengthen our spirit and develop a greater capacity to face, address, and allow God to heal our negative emotions and past pain by applying forgiveness to ourselves and others. The storage closet of hurt feelings begins to empty out, as we seek and follow God's will and stay rooted in the Word. The triggers have less to activate in us, so we are not responding with the same levels of fear and stress. Instead, we have trust and faith. We become less selfish, and less seeking of gratification through mood alteration. We become more selfless - more interested in others - and how we can contribute to their well-being instead of taking what we think we need to feel good inside.

When we are operating in the peace of the spirit, we don't develop internal triggers as often, either. Blood sugar levels are more even and steady, because we care about what we eat and we try to balance our protein, carbohydrate and fat so we stay energized and steady until the next meal. We sleep better, and make self-care a top priority. We find and face our strongholds, ask God to remove them, and keep new ones from forming by taking thoughts and purposes away captive unto the obedience of Christ. We don't activate harmful thoughts by acting on them. We turn to God and the Word instead. God gives us great strength through scripture, and through other believers, to rest in the peace of His spirit and to be free of strongholds and triggers that can turn thoughts into harmful actions.

In Diagram 4, we see that stress compounds create the desire to engage in behavior to alter stress and produce feel-good compounds. If we choose to lead the thought away captive unto Christ, we choose a God-focused activity like reading the Word, or prayer. If we choose a harmful behavior, like eating, overspending, drugs, or addictive relationship behavior, we activate the cycle that produces short-term gratification, followed by guilt, shame, remorse and fear, thereby triggering the release of more stress, and more attempts to change the feeling again by seeking fleshly pleasures. These cycles reinforce power on the activity and create strongholds, or neural pathways, that are the ruts in our soul that we dig deeper each time.

God's Word and prayer have the power to resurface the road in our soul. The ruts that we have dug, through our patterns of stress and then temporary release, can be filled by healing the hurt emotions and breaking down the strongholds. We become different people on the inside, and the influence of the Holy Spirit on our thoughts and behaviors flows freely when it isn't barricaded by stronghold fortresses. Strongholds actually block the flow of information (Truth) into the soul from the Spirit. Strongholds wrap themselves around beliefs so that the Truth cannot penetrate through the mind regarding this area of thought. The stronghold is a proud and lofty thing, an argument that exalts itself against the knowledge of God.

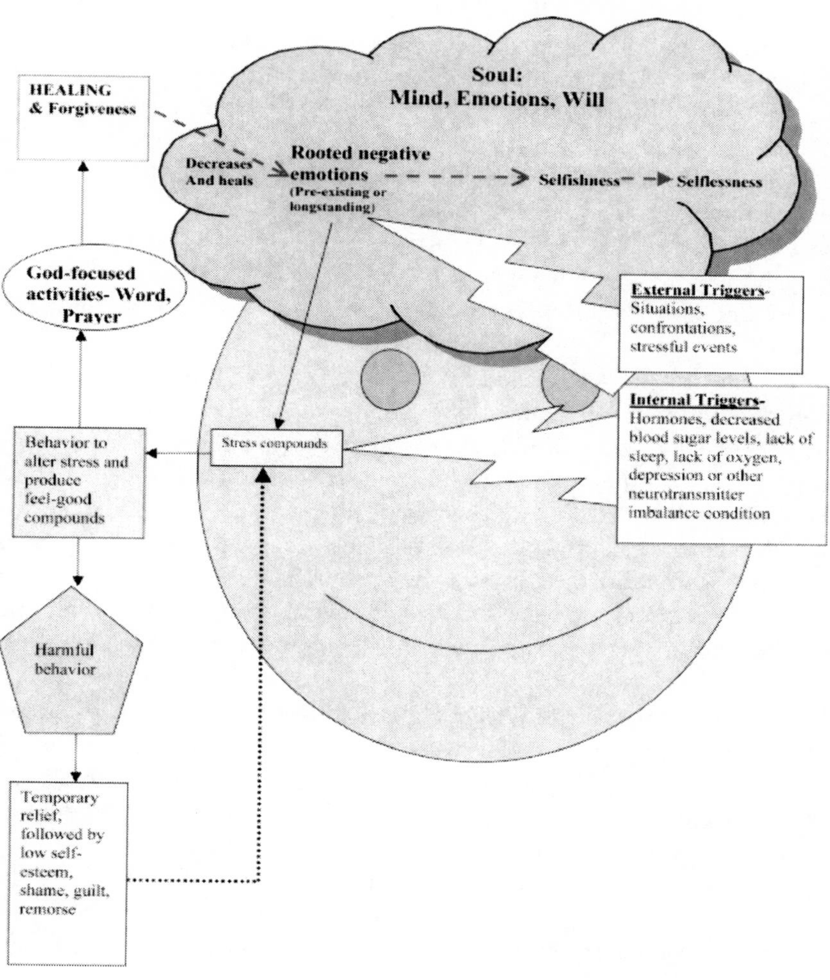

Mindful Eating

Thus far, we have dealt with strongholds that block the flow of the Spirit. We have begun the journey of emotional healing through the Holy Spirit, to be free of stress and other harmful thoughts that can create body chemistry that leads to weight gain, low energy, and reliance upon food to change our mood.

We now need to address lifestyle issues. I used to work with a man who used the phrase "that's the tail wagging the dog" to describe situations where the proper priority is out of perspective, and the less important things are ruling over the most important. Many people do this with their eating habits.

We can't treat food as an incidental necessity that we grab on the run. When you do this, your body doesn't register satisfaction from the meal the way that it does when you sit down and slowly and mindfully chew your food, and enjoy a pleasant meal. Mindful eating is a great exercise to try, to introduce the realization that **it takes 20 minutes to reach satiety**, whereby the stomach tells the brain it has had something to eat, and it is full. This twenty minute period doesn't shorten if you gobble down five pieces of pizza. It still takes twenty minutes. So in that period of time, you can do a lot of damage! You could eat a whole day's worth of calories in less than twenty minutes, and not be aware that you are stuffed until AFTER the time has passed.

You can also feel very dissatisfied with your food and want more, if you eat quickly and still have quite a few minutes left. I have witnessed this at a hospital where I work with developmentally delayed adults. They get very excited when it is time to eat, and I have several patients who eat so quickly, they would choke to death if our dietary department didn't grind all of their food. They have such a yearning to feel satisfied that they will literally cram food into their mouths without properly swallowing. The faster they eat, the more dissatisfied they are when the food is gone. I eat with my patients and try to help them slow down, so they will be more satisfied (and safe when eating).

One strategy that helps us slow down is to drink water before the meal. As the liquid reaches the stomach, it helps us begin to register the inflow of nourishment. Another good practice is to begin your meal with a salad that is designed to give you a large volume of food without the calorie-dense toppings like full-calorie salad dressings, nuts, cheese, bacon, ham, or other meats. The best type of salad to begin to fill your stomach and tick off the minutes to reach satiety starts with spinach or mixed field greens (the darker salad green varieties are more nutritious), topped with other veggies like carrots, broccoli, sliced zucchini, mushrooms, water chestnuts, pea pods, and other non-starchy vegetables. You might want to add a few olives (3-4, these are high calorie) and some banana peppers for kick. Use the low-calorie dressing.

Some people actually trigger their cravings for more starchy foods when they begin eating restaurant bread before the meal. If you are one of those folks who can sit and eat the whole basket of bread (and you know who you are!), it is best to avoid it. Either ask the server not to bring it to the table, or put it at the opposite end of the table, by others in your party who don't have the same temptation.

Continue drinking water throughout your meal. These suggestions can put you in better control when dining out, so you aren't eating a huge plate of food when half the plate would have sufficed.

Keep in mind that we live in a society of food ABUNDANCE. We are not worried about finding food. On the contrary, we need to be very selective to AVOID food that we don't need. This can be a big problem for people who work at places where co-workers regularly bring snacks, desserts, doughnuts and other fattening treats for everyone to enjoy. I have learned the hard way that most of this junk isn't worth the calories it puts in my body. I try to consider my food intake throughout the day in terms of how much I have eaten, and if I am within my calorie budget. I don't carry a calculator- there is no need to be so precise! Once you learn the most expensive types of food, calorie and fat-wise, you can make informed choices, too. I usually am not willing to eat a less satisfying supper so I can eat a stale fried doughnut filled with fluff that tastes like whipped shortening. Worse, I have discovered that when I indulge in these sugary foods, I WANT MORE. It may come up later that night as a craving for cookies, or candy, but I have seen the effects enough to decide it is NOT WORTH IT.

This is one of the ways I believe the enemy sets us up to destroy ourselves from the inside. It is common nowadays for adults and children to skip breakfast, eat a vending pastry or a pop-tart and a soda mid-morning, and then grab a fast-food lunch. They may also order a sugary caffeine-filled drink from the local coffee house, at 300-450 calories a cup. Then, in the afternoon, they are really tired and need energy, so they grab another soft drink and candy bar. Supper might be pizza or a burger and fries.

This description might not sound harmful, but let me assure you, the beginning of the problem started at breakfast. The body needs to begin the day with a nice breakfast with protein, good quality fat, and carbohydrates. We will discuss these particulars more in the third section of the book. When you feed on sugar at breakfast, like a pop-tart or a pastry, the food item is quickly burned and turned into blood sugar by the body. This sends your energy level (blood sugar) soaring, but also requires that your body secrete a lot of insulin to bring the energy back down to normal by getting that energy inside the cells of the body where it can be burned off. This high circulating insulin is now considered to be a precursor of most major disease, by the way.

The bad news is, when the body has to put out a lot of insulin in response to a heavy blood sugar load, it can actually bottom out your energy afterward, so that you are even MORE tired than before. This is what the media now likes to call the "energy rollercoaster", the "sugar highs and lows", or a sugar "crash". You would think that with all the media attention focused on this problem, people would have changed their eating habits. Hopefully you see now, through the work we've done so far, that all the knowledge in the world won't change who you are and what you do. Christ changed who you are through His work on the cross. By seeking deliverance from strongholds and emotional bondage, you are free to use this knowledge about nutrition to actually make a difference, instead of buying a diet that tells you every bite of food to eat for two weeks and then thinking that will change you.

Back to the sugar crash. Once your blood sugar bottoms out, you feel tired and hungry again and you are reaching for another fix. You have probably learned that caffeine gives you energy, and wow, think of putting caffeine and sugar together- now that's a powerful boost. Caffeine causes the adrenal glands to secrete adrenaline, a stress hormone that makes you more alert, but also has an unpleasant effect of wiping you out when you use it for the sake of feeling more awake throughout the day. So you go through the coffee shop drive-thru and order a large mocha chip drink. Think of this as a chocolate-filled doughnut in a cup, with a shot of caffeine added. And it's only 10:00 am.

The fast food lunch introduces a new twist to the chemical mess we're making inside our body. A high-fat burger and fries set off brain chemicals like galanin, that trigger the desire for even more high-fat foods. This meal would make you feel satisfied for several hours because it would stay in your stomach longer, due to the high fat content. But as the meal wears off, the tiredness sets in again, and off we go to the vending machine for a candy bar and a coke. When we begin eating sweet foods, like chocolate, ice cream or cake, our body levels of endorphins rise. Endorphins are feel-good chemicals that are your body's natural morphine. As these levels rise, the urge sets in to eat more and more of the sweet food. It is interesting that endorphin levels don't rise in response to eating vegetables, or other natural foods. Be careful though, there are some concentrated but "natural" sugar sources, like maple syrup and honey, that are better for you than table sugar but do raise blood sugar levels and can trigger the effect of craving. I recommend Stevia instead, a natural, plant-based sweetener that does not raise blood sugar and is virtually calorie-free.

This eating scenario was not designed to make you feel bad about yourself, if you do any or all of these things. It is to show you that there are forces at work that you may not be aware of, in the blood and brain chemistry, that become *the tail wagging the dog* if you don't pay attention to what you bring into your body. The overall effect of doing these things day after day is an increased risk of diabetes, weight gain, and adrenal fatigue. The weariness and lack of energy can block your inspiration from the Holy Spirit, when you are just "too tired" to read the Bible, or minister to a friend in Christ. Your prayer time may be cut short when you don't feel well. The enemy delights in seeing us wiped out and defeated.

Are you eating breakfast daily? What do you eat, and how soon do you eat after you awaken?

____

____

____

Do you eat snacks at mid-morning or in the afternoon? What do you eat? How often?

____

____

____

____

Here's another eating scenario that may be familiar to many people. You wake up and skip breakfast altogether, because you don't have time and you feel that when you eat breakfast, you are often hungrier than if you didn't eat it. So you go along on coffee or some other beverage until lunch, and you grab something small. You feel pretty good about not having overeaten, because you know you haven't had much in the way of fat or calories.

When supper rolls around, you finally sit down with your family and eat a decent meal. You eat reasonable portions of a nutritious, balanced meal and maybe even a small dessert. Life is great, and your self-control in having only eaten one "real" meal and minimal light food earlier is proof positive that you are going to win at the weight game, once and for all.

Around 8:00 pm, the family is ready to sit down and watch television, and Dad wants a snack. After you allow yourself a small handful of chips, you settle down to watch your show. Those chips start to seem pretty harmless, considering how little you've eaten today. Another handful won't hurt. Now the ice cream sounds tempting, so maybe a small dish isn't going to hurt anything.

As the evening winds down for bed, you're still hungry. Once the kids are off to bed, it's time for one last trip to the kitchen to see what else might put the perfect finish on a day of pleasant, enjoyable eating.

Wow. This mentality stacks a huge number of the fattiest calories of the whole day at night, after 6:00 pm, when you will be sleeping in a few hours rather than having the opportunity to burn off what you've eaten. Research has shown that eating the same number of calories earlier in the day can lead to weight loss, as opposed to eating most of the same number of calories in the evening, which causes weight gain. While you sleep, your metabolism slows to its' lowest burning ability of the whole day. This isn't the time to load in a bunch of calories. Really, the less you eat at least four hours before bedtime, the better.

The other struggle we face is our feast-or-famine genetic hardwiring. Remember in the beginning of this book, we discussed that our bodies cue us to keep eating, once food is available, because we descended from tribes who had to go for longer periods without food. When they did eat, they stored extra fuel in their bodies as fat, and their appetites drove them to eat plenty, when it was available.

When you go without breakfast, you have deprived your body of food for all of the hours while you sleep, plus the hours until you eat again. Your genes send signals that the tribe isn't killing anything, so your appetite dies down. The small salad or quick bite at lunch was only enough food to convince your genes that someone in the tribe who felt sorry for you might have slipped you a few berries.

So when supper hit, your genes were screaming, "feed me!" You ate, and you continued to eat all evening, until bedtime. This is the typical experience of dieters who think they are beating the system if they only eat a small number of calories before supper. On the contrary, we need to live by the old adage, "eat breakfast like a king, lunch like a prince, and supper like a pauper."

The Economics of Food: The Nutritional Cost of our Choices

Imagine if you were given a budget of $160 a day to spend at the mall. This might seem like a generous arrangement, but if you go to an expensive clothing store and begin picking up blouses and skirts without looking at the price tags, you will probably blow your budget very quickly. Now imagine that you disregard the cost, because you are so driven by want that you pay no attention to the total price of the items you selected. When you get to the register, you tell the clerk to put the amount you owe on credit. You don't bother to ask how much you went over your budget.

As you go deeper into debt, you notice that your finances are in serious trouble. You are now addicted to this lifestyle, shopping at fine stores and wearing expensive clothes that you cannot afford. You feel entitled to do this, because you see others spending the same way, and they don't question the cost. Sometimes they moan about having to "cut back", but they still shop at the finest stores and don't compare prices, or question if they really need the things they are buying. What does this have to do with eating, you ask?

Many Americans behave the same way with food as I have described in the example above. We each have a unique number of calories that our body requires each day to keep us at our present weight. If we eat fewer calories than we need, we lose weight. If we exceed our calorie budget, we gain weight. The effects are cumulative, just like spending money. Instead of accumulating debt, we get fat. **Fat is excess caloric intake, manifested on our bodies.**

But just as you can learn to be financially responsible, you can also learn to manage your eating. Most men and young, active women will lose weight gradually, or maintain a healthy weight, if they stay between 1800-2200 calories a day. Some will require more calories, depending upon exercise and other physical movement, and age. Younger athletic men may need 2400-2800 calories or more per day. Men over the age of 40, who are not athletic, will lose weight more quickly on 1600 calories daily.

Women over 40, with small amounts of exercise, can gradually lose weight by eating 1400-1600 calories daily. Eating much below 1400 calories can create a deprivation mentality that can result in excess hunger and cravings.

Once you know your calorie budget, you should familiarize yourself with the caloric cost of various foods. For a surprising list of good and bad calorie bargains, see Diagram 5. In general, convenience foods and fast foods tend to be very high in calories. The more "flavor" they tout - cheese, sauces, breading, seasonings, dressings - the higher the calories, fat, and salt. Learn to enjoy and appreciate simple foods, like steamed vegetables, fresh fruit, salads, baked or broiled meats and seafood. Try seasoning foods with lemon, pepper, wine, vinegar, mustard, and herbs. Begin making different choices in where you eat, and more importantly, eat at home, where you can control how the food is prepared!

Most desserts are high in calories, but there are exceptions. Popsicles are small and tend to be lower in calories than ice cream. Fruit ice, sherbet, and frozen yogurt are also alternatives to ice cream, if less than 90 calories per half cup. For an almost calorie-free dessert, try sugar-free Jello with Cool Whip topping. Sugar-free pudding is another low calorie option. Watch out for sugar free cookies and snack cakes because the calorie content is usually high in these items.

Does this mean you should never be able to enjoy favorite meals, like fried chicken, macaroni and cheese, or rich desserts, like cheesecake? No way! We should eat and enjoy food, because it is a pleasurable activity that God has created for us to appreciate. But as we learn the impact of different types of food on our health and energy levels, we will begin to realize what meal choices are beneficial, and which should be limited to a smaller percent of our overall eating.

I advocate the 80:20 guideline - that eighty percent of what we eat should be considered healthy food, or reasonably so, and twenty percent can be purely for pleasure. If health problems exist like diabetes or high blood pressure, it is wise to spread out our more indulgent food to be a much smaller part of a healthy meal, so that the food can be a treat, and not an entire meal.

For example, if I have high blood pressure and I love to eat salty potato chips, I would first want to know what a realistic daily intake of sodium should be, likely around 2000 milligrams of sodium daily.

As I learn which foods are high in sodium and which are low, I would enjoy a meal of lower sodium foods and include a reasonable portion of potato chips, based on what the food label says one serving should be. Generally, it will be about 15 chips. I will also see that this number of chips has about 240 milligrams of sodium, which is a manageable amount to take in without overdoing it. Had I eaten half the bag of chips, I would have consumed far too much sodium, taken along with the other food I would eat in a day's time.

But We Take Pride in Mama's Cooking!

Cultural eating styles are a delightful part of American society. Most major cities offer a variety of ethnic restaurants where everyone can taste and enjoy different foods. True, authentic ethnic meals will reflect the agriculture and tradition of their country of origin. For example, traditional Japanese food may include white rice, Bonito fish, seaweed, and pickled vegetables.

Researchers have demonstrated increased health problems when various cultures stray from their traditional diet staples and eat American-style fast foods and snacks. Any human being suffers when they eat too much corn syrup, hydrogenated (plasticized) fat, sugar, and chemical-laden foods, which dominate our food supply. A healthy, traditional American meal would be based on fresh, garden-grown vegetables, tree fruits like apples, fresh beef and milk, and maybe even a little bacon fat (gasp!) for flavor.

The small amounts of lard, bacon fat, real butter and high-fat milk that farming Americans once ate was efficiently metabolized in all of the physical labor it took to produce these foods, on the farm.

Nowadays, we sit at desks and type on computers, our children play video games indoors, and we have to schedule time to work out at a fitness center or take a walk around the block, to get any exercise at all.

We walk up and down supermarket aisles and purchase packaged, canned or frozen foods that are loaded with salt, preservatives, sugar, and saturated fat. The fiber content is very low, and the vitamin and mineral levels are minimal. Fake colorings and flavorings are added to make the food more desirable. Many of the predominating ingredients raise our blood sugar levels and demand our bodies to produce more insulin to assimilate the energy from these foods, which creates more inflammation in the body and leaves us feeling tired and drained.

Our dairy foods are processed, held on the shelves for weeks, and contain antibiotics and hormones which are fed to the cows to help them create more milk and meat, without regard for their comfort or care.

We stay hungry because we derive very little lasting nutrition from the synthetic stuff we drink and snack upon, and the main ingredients - sugar, fat, and salt - destroy our health over time.

Some cultures have suffered much higher rates of diabetes, cancer, obesity and high blood pressure, as a result of the destructive elements of the American diet being introduced into their lives and becoming the mainstay of their diet. The Pima Indians of Arizona maintained much of their traditional way of life and economy until the late 19th century, when their water supply was diverted by American farmers settling upstream. At that time, their 2,000-year-old tradition of irrigation and agriculture was disrupted, causing poverty, malnutrition and even starvation. The Pima community had to fall back on the lard, sugar and white flour the U.S. government gave them to survive. Presently, half of all adult Pima Indians have diabetes and 95% of those with diabetes are overweight. (From: The Pima Indians, Obesity and Diabetes, www. diabetes.niddk.nih.gov)

African Americans are at twice the risk for developing diabetes, and are at greater risk for heart disease, stroke and other cardiovascular diseases (CVD) than Caucasians. The prevalence of CVD in African American females is 44.7 percent, compared to 32.4 percent in white females (http://www.muschealth.com/heart/women/africanwomen.htm). African American men are at high risk of developing prostate cancer; one in five will be diagnosed with prostate cancer and one in twenty will die from it (http://www.cdc.gov/cancer/prostate/publications). These figures are much lower in other races and ethnic groups.

If we farmed and ate the fresh, nutritious versions of home-cooked meals, most African and Caucasian Americans would be able to enjoy traditional meals without the health risks. But unfortunately, we eat so much processed, synthetic, quick food, drinks and snacks throughout most of our lives, that the rich down-home meals we love just add insult to injury. Again, consider the 80:20 guideline. If the majority of our food choices were healthy and sound, the wonderful indulgent meals of fried chicken or ribs with home-baked pies and desserts wouldn't cause nearly the trouble they do now. They would have even less of a negative impact if we made some effort to use healthier ingredients in cooking and preparing these meals, took smaller portions of the most fattening items, and looked for ways to include more activity and exercise into each day. Then our down-home meals would become a treat, rather than an unhealthy lifestyle.

Part III

In the Body: Seeds Falling on Fertile Soil

Hopefully you haven't skipped the other two sections of the book, in an eagerness to get into the technical knowledge that you may have hoped for when you picked up this book. If we had planted the seeds of knowledge on shallow, rocky soil, they would have burned up quickly and died, before they could have taken root and grown. The awareness we sought from the Lord to recognize strongholds and rooted negative emotions was like pulling weeds. We have started to see our attitude and approach to eating more objectively, which will help plow the soil of the soul, and fertilize it so that what we now plant can grow strong. The sunlight of the Spirit can shine down into us and fill our mind, emotions and will, and come back out into the world through the words we speak, which become a barometer of our inner conditions. Jesus said, in Matthew 15:11: "*It is not what goes into the mouth of a man that makes him unclean and defiled, but what comes out of the mouth; this makes a man unclean and defiles him.*"

With the right focus on the inside, we make choices based on loving and caring for ourselves as the tabernacle of the Holy Spirit, rather than pursuing those things which gratify the flesh. *Those who are according to the Spirit and are controlled by the desires of the Spirit set their minds on and seek those things which gratify the Holy Spirit.* (Rom 8:5)

The Basics of Eating

Here are Some Simple Guidelines to Summarize Good Basic Nutrition Habits:

1. Always eat breakfast. Skipping it sets you up for overeating later in the day and fails to stoke up your metabolism to keep burning calories at a more efficient rate.

2. Eat with intention - don't cram something in while you are driving or doing something else. Stop what you are doing and deliberately focus on slowing down and enjoying your food.

3. Chew your food thoroughly and try to make the meal last for twenty minutes. It takes twenty minutes to feel full, whether you eat a salad in that time, or an entire pizza buffet.

4. Drink plenty of water. Water is a free lubricant that keeps our bodies functioning properly. We are often more dehydrated than we realize. You should be drinking 60-80 ounces of water a day, or more if you are athletic or sweat on your job. Staying hydrated keeps you thinking more clearly. Good hydration helps your skin to be healthier, and you will be less likely to feel hungry as often. Next time you think you are a little bit hungry, drink a bottle of water first and see if you feel satisfied. We sometimes mistake hunger for thirst.

5. Most people do better to eat every 4-5 hours. Three reasonable-sized meals and 2 small snacks are appropriate. We will discuss portion sizes and sample snack ideas later.

6. Eat a balance of protein, carbohydrate and fat at meals and at snacks. These three nutrients slow each other down, so their conversion to blood sugar (energy fuel) lasts longer and keeps you more satisfied. The major health benefit to this approach is that your blood sugar level stays even and doesn't spike, which helps prevent the development of diabetes, and minimizes diabetic symptoms in those who have the condition.

7. Balanced eating of carbohydrate, protein and fat at every meal and snack lessens the production of brain chemicals that drive you to want to eat more sugar or fat. Your mood and energy are much more stable and steady, and your overall intake of calories will usually be less.

8. Avoid sugary drinks like fruit juices, bottled fruit drinks, and Gatorade. These are NOT health foods, in most instances. They contain a lot of calories in the form of sugars, and can raise your blood sugar very rapidly. Learn to love water. Nothing makes you feel as hydrated and satisfied as drinking pure water. Crucify that soda or fruit drink habit.

9. Limit your intake of coffee shop drinks, unless you are willing to stick to the lower calorie choices. Starbucks makes a drink called a "tea misto", made from your choice of various flavors of tea steeped in a mixture of 50% water and 50% milk or soymilk. This drink only contains about 75 calories and is very tasty. They also offer an iced passion tea that is calorie free, to which you can add Splenda or your own Stevia. The Frappuccino Light is available but still contains about 240 calories for a medium-size, which is the same calorie content as a small order of McDonald's French fries.

10. Try to allow yourself at least four hours between supper and bedtime. A small snack before bedtime is fine, but a large meal any closer than four hours before bed is asking for fat storage during the night and indigestion in the morning.

11. Become aware of your salt intake. The first step is to stop salting your food. Realize that fast food is very high in salt, and all of the sauces and add-on ingredients like bacon and cheese only make it worse. Salt can elevate blood pressure and cause water retention. As you eat less salt, you lose your taste for it. Salty foods will not taste good to you if you maintain a low salt intake in your daily diet.

Putting it all Together into Meals

We have seen how the enemy can use God's circuitry to lead us into temptation when our body chemistry is out of balance. The circumstances that can create the kind of brain chemistry that makes fatty, salty, or sugary synthetic foods irresistible are:

- Stress - worry, fear, confrontations, financial insecurity, anxiety about one's appearance, working too much, no "down" time.

- Eating sugary foods or drinks without protein and fat to slow them down - The rapid, unchecked conversion of sugary foods or drinks into blood sugar can make us all feel good temporarily, but then our energy bottoms out, and we are either tired, or craving more sugar, or both!

- Eating sugary or fatty foods that stimulate dopamine and serotonin, making us feel relaxed and loved while we are eating them, but turning into cravings and remorse later. Remember those food strongholds that you identified in Section 1? The answers you wrote in that section may help you recognize some of the foods that stimulate YOUR neurotransmitters in a manner that leads you into overeating behaviors.

- Other moods that we wish to change—Who enjoys feeling lonely, depressed, frustrated, tired, bored, or unfulfilled? Some of us have found relief in food, but this fix is temporary and leads to more craving, guilt and shame over the amount of food eaten and the weight gained.

How can we keep our energy levels and brain chemicals stable to avoid falling into these undesirable eating patterns? Hopefully, in the other sections of the book you have identified some of your old patterns and have released some of the strongholds that triggered undesirable food behaviors. Now, to strengthen ourselves in the body by making the right food choices, we have to be aware of the three major components of food that we need to eat to create balance, at each meal and snack:

- Carbohydrates
- Protein
- Fat

We are going to take a good look at each of these three nutrients, to determine the best and worst choices in each category, and why it is so important to eat these TOGETHER, to create energy and blood sugar stability.

Aren't we Avoiding Carbohydrates?

Americans love to believe there are magic secrets to weight loss, just by doing something "new" like avoiding carbohydrates, or fats. These avoidance diets resurface every five years or so. What we have learned over the years is that there is no glory in trying to avoid one nutrient category. It creates an imbalance. God created food to provide a nice balance of protein, carbohydrate and fat. If He had wanted us to avoid carbohydrates, He wouldn't have made foods like grains, fruit, beans, potatoes, syrup, honey, and rice. Man came along and processed these foods, added concentrated sugary syrups to them, and packaged them. They became more fattening, and lost their fiber content. Most grain used for making bread is so stripped of its natural goodness that the manufacturers throw a few vitamins back into it and call it "enriched". They really should call it bleached and depleted, because this is what most bread (and pasta) has become.

Several years ago, a rating scale called the *glycemic index* was created to rate how quickly various carbohydrate foods turn into blood sugar, so we can prevent our blood sugar from shooting up or down too quickly in response to what we eat. This might sound like something only a diabetic needs to think about, but we all need to prevent those highs and lows, to keep from BECOMING diabetic. Many of us carry the genetic potential for diabetes. Current estimates are that one in four Americans is in an early stage of pre-diabetes and is already showing signs of not handling sugars well. Their baseline levels of blood sugar are higher than they should be. Elevated blood pressure and heart disease are part of the cluster of problems people develop along with diabetes.

Which foods are considered carbohydrates?

- Grains, like rice, wheat, barley, oats
- Starchy vegetables, like corn, peas, lima beans, soup beans

- Bread and breading on foods, pizza crust
- Cakes, pies, candy, sherbet
- Potatoes
- Snack chips
- Soups
- Pasta

Remember the 80:20 rule? Carbohydrates should not be avoided. Really, any of them can be enjoyed in the right amounts, but the key is to know which are healthier and should be included in the 80% of the diet that is healthy, and which should be reduced to the 20% of the diet that is saved for the more indulgent types of food.

The glycemic index rates carbohydrate foods relative to glucose, which is blood sugar. The higher the score, the faster the food turns into blood sugar. Most beans, whole grains and non-starchy vegetables have low glycemic index scores while sugars, refined grains made from flour, some fruits, and root vegetables have higher glycemic index scores.

There is no need to memorize the scores of foods on the glycemic index. The good news is that if we eat complex (less refined or processed) carbohydrates along with protein and fat at the same time, **they slow each other down in their conversion into blood sugar**.

I like to have people imagine that they have a magnifying glass and they are looking at the food in question up close. Think about breakfast cereal, for example. The surface of a rice krispie would be very porous, like a sponge, under your magnifier. A piece of bread would look the same way. These foods are so porous that your stomach acid and digestive enzymes can break these foods apart very rapidly and turn them into blood sugar. These foods would be very high on the glycemic index. Rice Krispies Cereal wouldn't be as healthy as a more solid, slower-to-digest cereal like All-Bran or Bran Buds.

Sugary sodas and fruit flavored drinks are the same way. There is really nothing to break down in the digestion of these liquids, so they are turned into blood sugar very quickly.

Pies, cakes, and cookies are all turned into blood sugar quickly in our bodies. These "fast" carbohydrates have very little fiber or protein to slow down their conversion into blood sugar. We call these types of carbohydrates "simple" or "fast" carbohydrates. Sweeteners like sugar and syrup are fast carbohydrates.

Slower-converting carbohydrates are better choices because they help stabilize blood sugar. Listed below is a table of best, moderate, and worst carbohydrate choices, and the appropriate portion size for one serving. **Fruits and fruit juices are also considered carbohydrates**. The list of fruit choices will follow the carbohydrate choices. Remember with fruit, fresh is best, then frozen. Canned fruit is next best, if packed in water. Avoid fruit canned in heavy syrup or even its' own juice, if you can find those that are water-packed. Dried fruit and fruit juice are very high in calories. Eat very small portions. Fruit juice servings should be limited to 4-6 ounces, which is HALF of a small coffee cupful. Dried fruit should be limited to a small handful.

BEST Carbohydrate Choices:			
Beans		**Seed Vegetables**	
Black beans	½ cup	Green peas	½ cup
Black eyed peas	½ cup	Corn	½ cup
Hummus	2 Tbsp	Mixed	
Dried beans, cooked	½ cup	vegetables	1 cup
(such as kidney, pinto)		Succotash	¾ cup
Garbanzo beans	½ cup		
(chickpeas)			
Lentils	½ cup		
Refried beans	1/3 cup		
Lima beans	2/3 cup		
Breads		**Potatoes**	
35-calorie, 5 net		New potatoes	½ cup
carbs per slice bread	2 pieces	(2 small)	
Lo-carb wrap bread		Sweet potato	1 small
tortilla (5 g net carb)	1 tortilla		
Pita bread	1 (1 ounce, or 6")		
Cereals and Grains		**Soups**	
All-bran cereal	½ cup	Choose reduced sodium soups for	
Bran buds	1/3 cup	blood pressure concerns, and to	
Old-fashioned	½ cup cooked	decrease water retention.	
Oatmeal		Read label to identify the portion size	
Pasta	½ cup	for 80 calories, equal to one starch serving.	
Barley	½ cup		
Bulgar	½ cup		
Buckwheat	1 ounce		
Snacks			
Light or lowfat popcorn	1½ cups		
Nutrition bar - check nutrition label - choose those with 150-175 calories			

Moderate Carbohydrate Choices	
These starch foods are not as supportive to health as the Best choices, but should be included in your meals in moderation:	
Grains	
White or whole wheat bread	1 slice
Couscous	¼ cup cooked
Millet	¼ cup cooked
Rice - basmati or brown rice	1/3 cup cooked
English muffin	½ muffin
Pretzels	½ cup
Animal crackers	8
Graham crackers	3 (2½ inch square)
Whole grain waffle	1
Cereals (3/4cup)	**Potatoes**
Bran flakes	White - 1 small, fist-size
Cheerios	Mashed - ½ cup
Corn Chex	
Cornflakes	
Cream of Wheat	
Muesli	
Nutri-Grain	
Special K	
Total	
Snacks	
Whole grain crackers, preferably	
low sodium:	
Nut Thins	12 crackers
Wasa Crispbread	2 slices
Ryvita Crackers	2
Worst Choices - limit these in your diet!	
Bagel	½ bagel
Hamburger or hot dog bun	½
Dinner roll	1
Saltine crackers	6
These count as a starch and a fat:	
Biscuit, 2 ½ inches across	1
Crackers, butter-type	6

Croutons	1 cup
French fried potatoes	2 ounces
Small muffin	1 (1½ ounces)
Pancake, 4 inches across	2
Popcorn, not low fat	3 cups
Sandwich crackers with	
cheese or peanut butter	
filling	3
Taco shell	2
Tortilla chips	10
Better Dessert Ideas	
Angel food cake	1 small slice
Fruit ice	½ cup
Sorbet	½ cup
Frozen yogurt	½ cup
Fruit Servings	
Remember, fresh is best, then frozen, or canned in water, then dried	
Apple, unpeeled	1 small (4 ounces)
Applesauce, unsweetened	½ cup
Apples, dried	4 rings
Apricots, fresh	4 whole (5.5 ounces)
Apricots, dried	8 halves
Apricots, canned	½ cup
Banana, small	1 (4.5 inches)
Blackberries	¾ cup
Cantaloupe, small cubes	1/3 melon (11 ounces) or 1 cup
Cherries, sweet, fresh	12 (3 ounces)
Cherries, sweet, canned	½ cup
Dates	3
Figs, fresh	1½ large, or 2 medium (3.5 ounces)
Figs, dried	1½
Fruit cocktail	½ cup
Grapefruit, large	½ (11 ounces)
Grapefruit sections, canned	¾ cup
Grapes, small	17 (3 ounces)
Honeydew melon	1 slice or 1 cup cubed
Kiwi	1 (3½ ounces)
Mandarin oranges, canned	¾ cup

Mango, small	½ fruit (5½ ounces) or ½ cup
Nectarine, small	1 (5 ounces)
Orange, small	1 (6½ ounces)
Papaya	½ fruit (8 ounces) or 1 cup cubed
Peach, medium, fresh	1 (6 ounces)
Peaches, canned	½ cup
Pear, large, fresh	½ cup (4 ounces)
Pears, canned	½ cup
Pineapple, fresh	¾ cup
Pineapple, canned	½ cup
Plums, canned	½ cup
Prunes, dried	3
Raisins	2 Tbsp
Raspberries	1 cup
Strawberries	1 cup (sliced)
Strawberries, whole	1¼ cup
Tangerines, small	2 (8 ounces)
Watermelon	1 slice, or 1¼ cup cubed

Lean, Mean Protein

Protein is an important nutrient to include at each meal. It slows carbohydrate so that it doesn't turn to blood sugar too quickly. It provides amino acids that the body uses for hormone production, wound healing, muscle rebuilding, and many other critical functions. Without adequate protein, our immune system becomes compromised and we are more susceptible to infections. However, most Americans eat much more protein than the body requires. The recommended intake for most adults is around sixty grams a day, but many Americans eat two to three times this amount. While this is usually not dangerous, it does reflect the sad disparity between our abundance of food and the poverty of third world countries that struggle to produce enough protein to keep their populations from becoming malnourished.

Protein is plentiful in our food supply, particularly in animal meats. Fast food offers us a ready supply of protein from burgers, chicken, fish, cheese, and deli meat sandwiches. We also obtain protein from dairy food, eggs, nuts, and beans. Peanut butter is a good source of protein.

Vegetarians and meat eaters alike obtain adequate protein with very little effort. The key consideration with protein is to **watch the preparation and fat content**. Fatty meats, fried meats and breaded seafood have a higher fat content than their baked or broiled lean counterparts, so it is easy to gain weight and elevate your cholesterol levels with these foods. Examples of high fat meats include ribs, roast, organ meats, bacon, and dark meat chicken and turkey. Most fast food burgers are made from fatty meat. These, along with breaded fried fish, chicken, shrimp and other fried seafood, belong in that 20% "special indulgence" section of the diet. If you are eating fast food burgers, fish, and chicken more than once or twice a week, you are adding a huge amount of calories, salt and fat to your diet that may lead to weight gain and health problems.

Fat Phobia

I remember when low-fat diets were all the rage. Back in the 80's and 90's, Americans had the idea that if they ate only twenty grams of fat a day or less, they would lose vast amounts of weight, regardless of the number of total calories they consumed!

I am quite familiar with some of the low fat approaches. They worked well when people chose lots of vegetables, fruits and whole grains as the basis of their diets, along with lean chicken, beef, pork and seafood. Everything was baked or broiled, never fried. One weight loss program of this era told clients that drinking regular, full-sugar soft drinks was acceptable, as well as desserts like jelly beans, because they are FAT FREE. How many of us ate boxes of low fat cookies, thinking we would lose weight?

The truth is, if we eat reasonable quantities of healthy fat sources at each meal, we are improving our satiety, and are less likely to feel hungry than when we avoid fat. The fat slows down how fast the stomach empties the meal, and slows the conversion of the food into blood sugar. We get a nice, slow, steady, even release of blood sugar when fat and protein work together to slow carbohydrates down. Add a complex carbohydrate source with fiber, like a fresh apple or steel-cut oatmeal, and you have created the best combination of foods to sustain your energy.

Healthy fats include olive oil, canola oil, fish oil and deep sea fish, nuts and seeds, avocados, and olives. Less healthy fats are those found in processed foods - that famous line in the ingredient label that says, "may contain one or more of the following: Cottonseed oil…" and fats that are found in animal foods. This would include higher fat percentage milk, like whole or 2%, fatty meats like organ meats, bologna, bacon, sausage, dark meat chicken and turkey, and high fat cheeses. Fat sources that are solid at room temperature, such as shortening and lard, are very unhealthy. The unhealthy fats promote inflammation, worsen cholesterol levels, and increase the risk of heart disease.

Portion Sizes

How much is the "right amount" of food? Restaurant portions have gotten larger over the years, and fast food super-sizing is a way of life. We need to step back and look at the portion sizes that are recommended by health experts:

Food Item	Portion Size	Reference Point
Cheese	One ounce	• Four dice • A wrapped single slice (as sold prepackaged)
Meat	Three ounces	• A cassette tape • A deck of cards • The palm of your hand • A checkbook
Fruit	One piece	• Fist-sized
Potatoes	One small	• Fist-sized
Beverages	8 ounces	• A clenched fist, turned sideways
Beverages-Juices	4 ounces	• A half-cup is the size of what fits in your cupped hand • Plastic, single serve juice container with foil lid = 4 ounces
Vegetables	½ cup cooked	• The amount that fits in one cupped hand
Vegetables, fresh	1 cup raw	• The amount that fits in two cupped hands
Pancake	One pancake	• A Compact Disc
Fats	One teaspoon	• Size of your thumb tip
Pasta	One half-cup	• Size of half a baseball

How do we put these portions together at meals? A typical meal plan of 1200-1400 calories would provide the following number of servings at each meal/snack:

Breakfast:	Lunch:	Dinner:	Snack:
2 oz. meat	2 oz. meat	3 oz. meat	1 oz. meat
1 fat	1 fat	1 fat	0 fat
1 starch	2 starches	2 starches	1 starch
1 fruit	1 fruit	1 fruit	0 fruit
1 low fat dairy	0 dairy	0 dairy	1 dairy
	1 vegetable	1 vegetable	

For details about carbohydrate ("starch") choices, and fruit choices, see carbohydrate tables.

Self- Assessment Questionnaire

Let's take a moment to evaluate ourselves honestly now, in light of the information we have discussed about nutrition, the emotions, and our own eating patterns.

The following questions will help you consider your eating behaviors and characteristics. Your answers should remain personal and confidential. A scoring system will allow you to identify some of the strengths and challenges you may face, and raise your awareness of the presence of these behaviors.

1. When I am sad, bored, lonely, or stressed, I find that food makes me feel better.

a. False
b. True

2. I eat sensibly around others, but I make up for it when I get by myself:

a. No, I eat about the same way all the time.
b. Sometimes I overeat when I am alone, but not regularly.
c. I look forward to time alone to eat, when I can really have as much as I want, and whatever foods and snacks I want, and I sometimes feel strong guilt, shame and/or remorse about how I eat secretly, in private.

3. When I go out to eat, and there is bread on the table:

a. I can take it or leave it. If I eat it, I eat small amounts so I can enjoy my dinner.
b. I always eat the bread, and I have to be careful not to eat too much of it.
c. I eat the bread, and once I start I cannot stop. I ask for more bread if the restaurant will bring it.

4. **When I eat at fast food restaurants:**

   a. I rarely eat fast food.
   b. I consciously choose items that are lower in calories and try to eat healthy, which may include eating out several times a week.
   c. I sometimes order healthy, but may often choose whatever I feel like eating, which may be a burger and fries, and desserts fairly often.
   d. I eat whatever sounds good, and it usually includes large burgers or breaded chicken/fish and fries, and could include a milkshake or dessert. I eat this way at least 3 times a week.

5. **I skip breakfast:**

   a. Never - it is a very important meal for me, and I eat a balanced breakfast without leaning too much on sausage and bacon.
   b. Occasionally, but I do try to eat something in the morning.
   c. I eat fast food breakfast frequently.
   d. I eat toaster strudel, pop tarts, or doughnuts most mornings.

6. **I experience feelings of being tired in the afternoons:**

   a. Rarely or never.
   b. Occasionally, and I will try to eat nuts, or a healthy snack.
   c. Frequently.
   d. Frequently and I will drink a regular soda and/or eat candy or have caffeine to perk me back up.

7. **I sometimes eat to alleviate stress, boredom, sadness, or to otherwise change the way I feel.**

   a. Rarely or never.
   b. Occasionally.
   c. Frequently.

8. **I could possibly have issues with hormonal imbalance - I am female, between the ages of 40 and 60, and have experienced difficulty sleeping through the night (waking between 2-4 am for no reason), some hot flashes, and sugar cravings.**

   a. No.
   b. Maybe.
   c. Definitely.

If your answers are mostly from the "a" and "b" choices, then you will probably benefit from some fine-tuning and awareness in improving your current eating habits. If you have several "c" and "d" answers, you may have strong emotional eating patterns and may see a dramatic difference as you become more aware of them. Your deliberate choice to seek God for comfort, rather than food, will heal the hurts and soothe the emotional and physical imbalances that drive you to eat when you are really not physically hungry.

Just Tell Me What to Eat!

Most people who seek the advice of a dietitian really just want us to tell them what to eat.

I have spent years designing menu plans for clients based on their likes and dislikes, creating clever breakfast, lunch and dinner choices, with 1-2 snacks a day, staying within their personal calorie budgets, keeping in the range of 50% carbohydrate, 25% protein and 25% fat, or whatever percentages their metabolic characteristics dictated would be best. Then I would design a shopping list, with all the foods grouped in the order in which they would appear in the grocery store, for the clients' convenience. It seemed that the more I could think for them and do for them, the greater their chances of success. I'm sure by now you see the dysfunction in all of this.

God set us free from rigid dietary laws and rules. We need only be conscious and aware of the "cost" of various foods, like fast food meals, to make better decisions about how often we indulge in these special treats. They can't be viewed as daily purchases. Otherwise, we go into debt with our health. This can create financial debt, too, as we try various drugs and costly medical procedures to alleviate the stress on our bodies and improve our physical conditions.

We must remember that the key to this is progress, not perfection. Before I became a Christian, I specialized in the esoteric intellectualization of nutrition. Now, I see that intricate scientific facts about food such as antioxidant properties, fatty acid ratios, and mineral content won't compensate for the mistakes we make when the soul doesn't line up with the Spirit. The Spirit is always in the proper position, but the soul can sure get out of alignment, driving us to make poor choices and in some cases, trying to compensate with rigid diet practices that may include the use of supplements and health foods that make exaggerated health claims.

Remember that God is the Potter, and we are the clay. Have you ever seen clay mold itself? We can become so enthusiastic about using nutrients and supplements to control our health by changing the composition of the soil, while forgetting that God is Jehovah-raffa, our Healer. While it can be wise to include a multivitamin-mineral supplement daily to cover your nutrient needs if you don't meet them with food, it can be expensive and dangerous to consume large doses of vitamins and minerals. The body has ratios of these nutrients that it keeps in balance, and if you blindly take large doses of individual vitamins or minerals, you may do more harm than good.

To offer you a glimpse of some healthier meal ideas, I am going to share some food charts and menus. By no means am I advocating that you FOLLOW these menus. They are offered as learning tools, to model what a "balanced" meal would look like. I will also provide you with guidelines to consider at fast food restaurants, so that you can make better choices. Sometimes you will want to eat the higher fat, richer types of food. Today at my church picnic, I had a large plate of pork barbeque, creamy coleslaw, baked beans, and homemade dessert. I loved every bite. I even had two glasses of sweet tea. But tonight, I will eat a much lighter supper, probably around 6 p.m., and will continue painting walls in my house and obtain several hours of exercise in the process.

The whole idea behind this book is to meet you where you are and to show you how better health and nutrition are possible even if you eat meat, potatoes, bread, fast food, and dessert. Because let's face it - most of us do!

Best and Worst Calorie Bargains

We all have a calorie budget we need to stay within, to maintain weight. If we eat less than our budget, we lose weight. If we go over the budget, we gain weight. Most women need about 1400-1900 calories a day, and most men need about 2000-2400 to maintain a constant weight.

Some foods are expensive, in terms of the calorie content and your daily budget. Others are fairly low in calories and you may enjoy including them as treats, without the guilt. See if you are surprised by this list:

Worst Choices	***Bargains***
Regular soft drinks- one 16 oz bottle is 200 calories	Flavored waters- usually zero calories. You can make your own by adding lemon or a splash of fruit juice to bottled water.
Pancake syrup- 1 tablespoon contains 50 calories, and most people use about four tablespoons on their pancakes	Diet sugar free pancake syrup- ¼ cup of Atkins has zero calories
Regular bread- at 80 calories a slice, it is adds up fast.	Diet bread - at 35 calories a slice, it is a much better bargain!

Bologna and fatty lunchmeats- one slice is around 90 calories, and who eats just one?	Lean sliced deli meats- try the lower sodium products. 2 ounces fills the bread nicely, for only 45 calories.
Fruit drinks- large bottles of exotic, fruit-flavored drinks fill the coolers of most food mart stores. The average Sobe fruit drink, in a 20 oz bottle, provides 300 calories.	Sugar free fruit drinks are now available that provide about 40-60 calories in an 8 oz serving.
Fruit on the Bottom-style yogurt- many of these yogurts are as high as 240 calories per container.	Some of the better choices of low fat fruit flavored yogurts have only 90 calories per container.
Salad dressings - pay particular attention to fast food dressings, which may add 150 calories to the salad itself	Low calorie salad dressings are usually under 40 calories per tablespoon, and make wonderful marinades for meat and seafood.
Regular-fat cheese - one small slice has 80-100 calories.	Fat free cheese- only 25 calories per slice, and low fat cheese sticks are about 90 calories for the entire stick.
Coffee drinks - the typical flavored coffee drink can range from 300-500 calories.	Starbucks has a Frappuccino Light that comes in three flavors. The small size, no whipped cream or syrup topping, is about 150 calories.
Turkey meat products - beware of some of the turkey sausage and ground turkey burgers- if made with dark meat, they are as high as regular ground beef.	Choose white meat turkey products, which are substantially lower in calories than the full-fat versions.
Candy bars- most have about 240 calories	Ferrara Pan jawbreakers- tiny, hard round jawbreakers that have about 5 calories each, and last a long time if you don't bite them

Fast food baked potatoes- when loaded, some of these huge spuds are 400-500 calories! Campbell's	Soup- many varieties have only 100 calories per serving and can Healthy Choice brand, and be filling. Try Soup in Hand. Avoid cream soups.
	Fruit and Yogurt Parfait- when you have To eat something sweet from McDonald's, Try the SNACK SIZE fruit and yogurt Parfait, without the granola topping. It Is only 130 calories. Or the apple wedges, With one pack of caramel sauce, for 100 calories.

Diagram 5. Best and Worst Calorie Bargains. From www.eatwisely.org, Terri Lykins RD.

No More Excuses: WE EAT BREAKFAST!

By now, you understand why it is important to start the day with breakfast, so that your blood sugar stays level and your thrifty food genes don't subconsciously prompt you to believe that you are starving. There is no better way to lock yourself into an evening of non-stop snacking than to skip breakfast.

Choose one from each category to create a breakfast that will stay with you. Some suggestions include all three columns in one food choice. Considering that it can be as easy as drinking a canned supplement on the way to work, there is NO EXCUSE not to eat a balanced breakfast.

Carbohydrate	Protein	Fat
½ cup applesauce	3 strips bacon	(counts as protein & fat)
½ bagel	1 egg cooked any way	1 pat butter/margarine

1 English muffin	1 slice cheese	1 TBSP cream cheese
Nutrigrain or cereal bar	1 piece Canadian bacon	1-2 TBSP Flaxseed oil
1 container yogurt (counts as carb & protein)	1 scoop protein powder	Small handful pumpkin or sunflower seeds
1 cup cooked oatmeal	2 healthy sausage links	(counts as protein & fat)
2/3 cup dry cereal	8 oz. skim or 1% milk	(2% or more is also a fat)
1-2 pieces toast	1 TBSP peanut butter	(counts as protein & fat)
1 piece fresh fruit	15 nuts	(counts as protein and fat)
1 SMALL box raisins	1-2 cheese sticks	(counts as protein and fat
1 waffle	Atkins Drink in a Can	(counts as protein and fat)
Trail mix in small pack	(counts as all three columns)	
Hi-protein Slim Fast	(counts as all three columns)	
South Beach Bar	(counts as all three columns)	
Smoothie (1/2 c. frozen fruit, 6 oz. milk, 1-2 TBSP flax oil, 1 scoop protein - complete meal		

Sample Reduced-Calorie Menu Using Common Foods

Breakfast	**Lunch**	**Dinner**
2 scrambled eggs	2-4 oz. lean hamburger	4 oz. baked chicken
½ c. cooked oatmeal	1 medium baked potato	2/3 c. brown rice
1 small orange	1 c. tossed salad	½ c. green beans
8 oz. skim milk	1 packet diet dressing	½ c. peaches
Snack: 15 almonds and 1 mozzarella cheese stick		

Great Stuff to Keep Around the House

If I don't have fattening chips, cookies and candy bars around the house, I don't have to worry about eating them. I have learned that I do need to keep a nice variety of alternatives on hand, though, so I don't feel like I am missing out on fun food to eat. Sometimes we want to snack for the enjoyment of it, rather than to medicate feelings. Here are some of the foods that are lower in calories that work well as snacks and treats:

Fruit cups - individually wrapped in single portions, 55 calories each
Applesauce cups
Diet pudding cups
Diet Jello and whipped topping
Individual packets of almonds (100 calorie serving, will be marked on package)
Lowfat popcorn, smaller sized bags
100-calorie snack packs (these come in multi-pack boxes)
Fresh fruit
Flavored ice pops
Cheese sticks
Hummus with veggie chips
Small boxes of raisins
Gobstopper jawbreakers- eat slowly, and they are lower in calories than most other candies!
90-calorie yogurt
High fiber cereal and skim milk

Please note that if sugar and snack foods are your weakness, you would want to avoid the sweets and chips choices on this list. The diet Jello and pudding should not create cravings, and the most bullet-proof choices for you would be cheese, hummus, almonds, and popcorn.

Meals on the Go, That Won't go to Your Waistline

Not all fast food is unhealthy. Many of us who choose to eat meals away from home several times a week can stay within an ideal weight range by making choices that reflect a concern for eating healthier. This is only a partial listing of several types of restaurants, offered as a starting point to help you consider your alternatives.

Best Choices at:

Fast Food Seafood Restaurants

- Baked whitefish
- Baked potato with small amount of sour cream
- Green beans
- Corn on the cob, request no butter, or wipe it off
- Seafood salad with boiled shrimp or crab,
- Request lowest calorie dressing on the side

Family Dining Seafood Restaurants

- Baked, broiled or blackened seafood
- Kabobs are usually a good choice
- Avoid breads served before and during meal
- Avoid cream soups and sauces
- Asked for steamed veggies with NO butter

Deli/ Sandwich shops

- Sliced lean deli meats with less bread
- Fresh salads with deli meats, request lowest calorie dressing on the side
- Check nutrition brochure in the restaurant to find the lowest calorie choices. Some Subway locations offer a low-carbohydrate wrap, as a lower calorie alternative to bread.

Chicken Restaurants

- Salads w/fat-free dressings
- Grilled chicken breast sandwich, request no sauce. Use ketchup and mustard.
- Chicken soup
- Chicken salad sandwich on wheat bread

Burger/Roast Beef Fast Food Establishments

- Small plain burger, with ketchup and mustard, lettuce, tomato, pickle and onion
- Junior roast beef sandwich
- Small (kid size) fries
- Plain baked potato, request broccoli with no cheese, as a topping, and use fat free sour cream
- Plain salad, with low fat dressing on the side
- Salads with broiled chicken, not fried, dressing on side
- Small (6 piece) nuggets

- Snack-sized yogurt parfait (without granola topping, counts as 1 fruit, 1 milk)
- Animal crackers
- Apple wedges

Health Food Stores

- Soups made fresh daily
- Deli items - excellent use of tempeh and tofu
- Frozen foods can be heated and eaten in the store
- Salad bar
- Fresh sushi if available - cooked recommended
- Fresh veggie juices available

Chinese/Thai Restaurants

- Choose tofu dishes, vegetarian dishes, or those that contain white meat chicken or shrimp - best choices are on the "Diet" section of the menu, where they offer the sauce separately from the vegetables/ meat. Use less sauce than offered.
- Request plain white or brown rice
- Best soup choices are egg drop and hot and sour soup
- Choose light colored sauces
- Avoid fried items
- Summer rolls, with steamed wrappers
- Chicken or shrimp satay or skewers, limit use of peanut sauce

Steakhouses

- Choose a lean steak, like tenderloin
- Choose a baked fish or shrimp entrée
- Select a sweet potato if available
- Corn or green beans
- Tossed salad
- Salad bar - use less croutons, cheese, bacon, fried noodles; olives, nuts and seeds (unless counting them as a fat serving)

Taco Fast Food Restaurants

- Bean burrito
- Side order of Spanish rice
- Chicken soft taco with lettuce and tomato
- Side of refried beans

As We Go From Here...

I pray that this book furthers your courageous journey into healing, forgiveness, transformation, and better choices. The nutrition information was intentionally kept simple and practical, to reflect the type of food choices you can make on a daily basis. While it would be ideal for everyone to eat tofu, tempeh, fresh vegetables and fruit, quinoa and amaranth grains, and drink ten glasses of reverse-osmosis filtered water a day, the reality is that most people are choosing fast food, processed snacks, and high-calorie coffee drinks on a regular basis. Food has become a drug that we use for false energy, comfort, and release from stress. The side effects are weight gain, poor health, and a soul hunger that reinforces power on the enemy to destroy us from within.

God gave us a way out through Christ. The Holy Spirit transforms us and empowers us to act out of our Christ-nature, when we turn to God through prayer and the Word.

> *Now we have received, not the spirit of the world, but the Spirit who is from God, so that we may know the things freely given to us by God. Which things we also speak, not in words taught by human wisdom, but in those taught by the Spirit, combining spiritual thoughts with spiritual words. (1 Cor 2:12-13, New American Standard Bible)*

For more information, visit www.eatwisely.org

CPSIA information can be obtained
at www.ICGtesting.com
Printed in the USA
FFOW02n1605260617
37175FF